AF698021

A10200 178723

Columbia University

Contributions to Education

Teachers College Series

No. 772

AMS PRESS
NEW YORK

TEACHING NUTRITION IN BIOLOGY CLASSES

An Experimental Investigation of High School Biology Pupils in Their Study of the Relation of Food to Physical Well-Being

BY

N. ELDRED BINGHAM, Ph.D.

TEACHERS COLLEGE, COLUMBIA UNIVERSITY
CONTRIBUTIONS TO EDUCATION, NO. 772

A Lincoln School Research Study

BUREAU OF PUBLICATIONS
TEACHERS COLLEGE, COLUMBIA UNIVERSITY
NEW YORK
1939

Library of Congress Cataloging in Publication Data

Bingham, Nelson Eldred, 1901-
Teaching nutrition in biology classes.

Reprint of the 1939 ed., issued in series: Teachers College, Columbia University. Contributions to education, no. 772.
Originally presented as the author's thesis, Columbia.
"A Lincoln School research study."
Bibliography: p.
1. Nutrition--Study and teaching (Secondary)--United States. I. Title. II. Series: Columbia University. Teachers College. Contributions to education, no. 772.

TX364.B55 1972 641.1'07'1173 74-176565
ISBN 0-404-55772-4

Reprinted by Special Arrangement with Teachers College Press, New York, New York

From the edition of 1939, New York
First AMS edition published in 1972
Manufactured in the United States

AMS PRESS, INC.
NEW YORK, N. Y. 10003

Acknowledgments

THIS investigation is the result of the cooperative efforts of many individuals. The author is indebted to the members of his committee for their expert guidance, to other members of the Teachers College faculty for consultation and advice, to the members of the Commission on Evaluation in the Eight Year Study of the Progressive Education Association for aid in the development of the tests, to the Lincoln School of Teachers College for its participation and support, and particularly to the teachers in the nine other school systems who tried out the array of educational experiences on which this investigation is based.

Professors S. Ralph Powers, chairman, John R. Clark, Mary Swartz Rose, and Ralph B. Spence, advisers for the study, have been most stimulating and helpful. They have given advice throughout the investigation, especially in regard to its relation to science education, its relation to general educational procedures, the scientific accuracy and social worth of the materials developed, and the educational research techniques employed. Much credit is due Professor Rose for her guidance in the selection and organization of content and experiences for use in teaching nutrition in biology classes.

Professor Lester Dix has been generous in allowing the writer the freedom of experimentation in the Lincoln School of Teachers College. Miss Jane Weber and Miss Bertlyn Bosley aided in teaching.

The author wishes to acknowledge the counsel of Dr. Gertrude H. Hildreth, Dr. Louis Raths, Professor Percival M. Symonds, and Dr. J. Wayne Wrightstone in the construction of the tests. Professor Irving Lorge has given invaluable aid in the selection and use of statistical procedures.

The twelve teachers in the several schools who found time, in the midst of heavy schedules, to participate in this investigation have contributed greatly to the findings secured. The intimate comparisons of actual school practices in the different schools prevent personal acknowledgment.

Valuable assistance was given by Miss Maude Kavanaugh, who helped in the compilation of the data, by Mr. Kenneth Hitch, who made many of the statistical calculations, and by Miss Eva Moore, who read the manuscript editorially.

To his wife, Marjorie Heath Bingham, the author is most indebted for her critical analyses and constant inspiration throughout the study.

N. E. B.

Contents

TEACHING NUTRITION IN BIOLOGY CLASSES

CHAPTER I

Introduction

As MAN has migrated from the farm to the city, he has had to depend more and more on others to produce the foods he consumes. Farming has become increasingly specialized as more of the products are grown or raised for ultimate consumption in distant cities. Manufacturers have found new ways to refine, preserve, and market foods. In some instances, essential food nutrients have been removed in the refining process. In other instances, seasonable foods have become staple throughout the year as a result of improved methods of producing, storing, and marketing. Today the grocer's shelf is filled with standard brands of countless varieties and forms of foods. Current magazines carry advertisements urging the consumer to buy this and that brand because of some real or imagined reason. These advertisements always stress the nutritive and health promoting properties, but it is unbelievable that the advertisers are prompted by such an altruistic motive. What is the consumer to do to be sure that he selects those foods which adequately meet his needs? He must select wisely from a far wider variety of products than ever confronted his ancestors.

Remington, who is a professor of nutrition, convincingly develops the thesis "that dietary instinct (upon which so many of us depend for our choice of food) is a distrust for the unknown, for those things of unfamiliar taste, and nothing more." [1] He summarizes his study as follows: "I have tried to set forth that the dietary instincts or habits of man are an outgrowth of certain *mores* which had their origins in the beginnings of tribal life, and were later influenced in their development by religion, by geographical habitat, by climate, by commerce, by modern industrial and inventive genius, and by advertising. I have shown that food likes and dislikes are taught in child-

[1] Remington, R. E., "The Social Origins of Dietary Habits," *Scientific Monthly*, Vol. XVIII, Sept., 1936, pp. 193-204.

hood, and though they may be slow to change, they do change as influenced by the factors mentioned above, and that dietary instinct is only a distrust for the unknown or for those articles of provender for which we have not acquired familiarity. The contributions of chemistry and physiology to our knowledge of nutrition, valuable as they may be to the livestock industry, have up to this time played a very minor part in directing the eating habits of the human species."[2]

Furthermore, the recent developments in the science of human nutrition are of such importance that they offer abundant rewards in human welfare. Sherman maintains that "In our understanding of the processes of life, perhaps the three greatest advances of the past hundred years have been, first, the establishment of the general principle of evolution with the subsequent working out of its genetic 'mechanism'; second, the discovery of the widespread existence and activities of bacteria and the development of the germ theory of infectious diseases and the science and techniques of sanitation; third, and latest, the development which for convenience we refer to as the newer knowledge of nutrition and of the nutritional characteristics of foods."[3] Sherman also stresses the returns in health to be gained by a careful consideration of foods:

"Present knowledge of nutrition and food values plainly shows the way, first to the avoidance of nutritional deficiencies, and then to the attainment of higher levels of health than we would otherwise enjoy. . . .

". . . it is quite conceivable that in the simple matters of the daily choice and use of foods lies our most important and practicable opportunity to build for the efficiency and happiness both of our lives and of the lives of those who are growing up under our care. . . .

". . . the option which the newer knowledge of nutrition offers is the option of a longer lease of healthier life, of an earlier and longer prime of life, of more buoyant health thruout the whole life cycle, as a result of taking a larger proportion of the needed calories in the form of protective foods."[4]

Sherman summarizes the experiments conducted in his own laboratory from which the above predictions are made: "Strictly quantita-

[2] Remington, *op. cit.*
[3] Sherman, Henry C., *Food and Health*, p. 1.
[4] *Ibid.*, Chap. XIX, pp. 185-187.

tive experiments with large numbers of [rat] families continuing through successive generations . . . showed that this same improvement in an already adequate diet (1) expedited growth and development, (2) resulted in a higher level of adult vitality as shown by several criteria, and (3) extended the average length of adult life, or improved the life expectation of the adult." [5]

That this expressed insight is not gained through the study of biology in high schools can be seen by a cursory examination of leading textbooks. With but one or two exceptions one can safely say that the material on human nutrition is so obsolete or unrelated to true pupil needs that it can not possibly function to any considerable extent in their daily lives.

Rose argues that "No one can be expected to exercise voluntary control over his diet or to undertake the task of training himself to eat unliked or new foods, unless he really believes that health is worth while to him personally, and that food will make a difference in some way that vitally touches his ambition." [6]

Much could be said concerning the interest shown by adolescent boys and girls in any factor which affects their rapidly maturing bodies. Social factors make them increasingly prone to scorn adult-imposed conventions. They tend to discard accustomed patterns of behavior and experiment in every conceivable manner. Their experiments in food, usually in the form of indulgence, do not yield results immediately, hence they are likely to draw conclusions that the old well-established health habits they have been following are valueless.

Roberts, who has had long experience in studying the teaching of nutrition to boys and girls, ably summarizes these points concerning high school boys and girls when she writes: "The tendency to challenge childhood teachings and practices is strong, as is also the urge for investigation and adventure. These urges can be utilized to set the students to working out for themselves the answers to their own personal as well as related community health problems. . . . There are health needs, moreover, in adolescence itself. The profound physiological changes which occur during this period, the

[5] Sherman, Henry C., *Nutritional Improvement in Health and Longevity,* Carnegie Institution of Washington, Supplementary Publication No. 25, Aug. 15, 1936, p. 4.

[6] Rose, Mary Swartz, *Teaching Nutrition to Boys and Girls,* p. 1.

acceleration in growth, the maturing of the reproductive system, and the development of the sex function, together with all their accompanying mental, emotional, and social implications, all entail new health problems and call for a vital type of education for healthful and wholesome living. . . . The increased demand of the adolescent for independence and his reluctance to accept the say-so of his elders require that he be given both before and during this time, such training as will enable him to be safely trusted with the management of his own program of living. . . . It should be kept in mind, furthermore, that the majority of high-school students will go out shortly to establish homes of their own, and that the education given them now for their own guidance may soon be put into practice in the rearing of their own children." [7]

There is such universal agreement among educators as to the importance of including in the curriculum those items which serve as a basis for living in accordance with practices most conducive to enduring health that little need be said from this standpoint. The investigator sees justification for the study in the objectives of general education, and more specifically in those of science education. In other words, the demands of adolescent boys and girls for accurate information on matters related to their personal health spurred the writer to undertake the study. That an adequate knowledge of matters related to one's health is considered one of the general objectives of education is shown by the following quotations.

The Commission on the Reorganization of Secondary Education stated that "the main objectives of education are: (1) health, (2) command of the fundamental processes, (3) worthy home membership, (4) vocation, (5) citizenship, (6) worthy use of leisure, and (7) ethical character." [8] The same Commission issued a report in which they stated that "science instruction is especially valuable in the realization of six of these objectives; namely, health, worthy home membership, vocation, citizenship, worthy use of leisure, and ethical character." [9] The treatment of health in science courses was emphasized in its relation to personal and community problems.

[7] Roberts, Lydia, *Nutrition Work with Children*, pp. 418 and 426.

[8] *Cardinal Principles of Secondary Education*, United States Bureau of Education Bulletin, 1918, No. 35, pp. 10-11.

[9] *Organization of Science in Secondary Schools*, United States Bureau of Education Bulletin, 1920, No. 26, p. 12.

The Committee on the Teaching of Science believes that "The maintenance of proper standards of health through control of causes of ill health is a responsibility of the individual and the community. An aim of the schools is to impart to children such instruction as will enable them to maintain bodily vigor. In meeting this responsibility attention should be focused upon three objectives: (1) the formation of health habits, (2) the imparting of health information, and (3) the development of a health consciousness. . . .

"Information raises health habits to the level of consciousness and makes them meaningful, and information provides the background which is the basis for intelligent action. . . .

"The citizen needs an appreciation of what health means to him and to the community. A health consciousness may be developed from the recognition of the comforts of the race that have come as a result of continuous progress in the control of ill health. A health consciousness, on a proper foundation of understanding, induces an obligation to carry forward programs of activity designed to protect the welfare of the group." [10]

With the rapid development of general science and general biology courses in the secondary school curriculum, hygiene, physiology, and other isolated health courses have been largely eliminated. Biology and general science have to a fair degree assumed the responsibility for education in the control of disease, but they have been slow in assuming the much needed role which would aid pupils in intelligently selecting and controlling their diet by making use of the newer knowledge of nutrition. Where should this instruction be furnished in the secondary school?

Evidence that a great deal of the responsibility for health instruction in our secondary school rests with the general science and biology teachers is gained from Cairns' study:

"There is need for better selection and better organization of instructional content. Time which could be used to advantage in teaching essentials is too often wasted in the teaching of non-essentials. . . .

"Health instruction which fails to teach the fundamentals fails to function in health promotion. This failure is largely due to the fact

[10] National Society for the Study of Education, *Thirty-first Year Book,* Part I, "A Program for Teaching Science," pp. 30-31.

that teacher-prejudices rather than scientific information determine health instruction. . . .

"The responsibility for health instruction is not always carried by those who should assume the major portion; that is, by the teachers of the fundamental sciences, who have the time and the facilities. . . .

"The chief responsibility for health instruction should not be placed on the physical education departments. They have other objectives than health education and cannot take the time from their activity programs to give pupils the scientific background necessary for intelligent health practices. Any attempt to assume this responsibility by groups other than those prepared to teach the underlying principles and having laboratories where pupils may have first-hand experience, results in dogmatic instruction. . . .

"The survey [Cairns] shows, then, that except for physiology, biology and general science include more of the essentials of health instruction than any other subject. This would seem to indicate that biology and general science, since they are more widely offered than physiology, are best able to carry the major responsibility for health instruction. There is need, however, to put more emphasis on human biology and physiology." [11]

To summarize, the selection of one's diet is much more complicated now than it was a generation ago. The science of nutrition has developed rapidly during the past few decades, yet little use of this knowledge is now being made by the general populace. Recent discoveries indicate that the general level of health can be raised by attention to diet. Because health is one of the major objectives of education and because adolescents are actively interested in their own welfare, it is important that they receive adequate instruction concerning the relation of food to physical well-being. Such instruction is not now generally given. Research studies indicate that this instruction may well be placed in biology classes. Related material as now presented in most biology textbooks is obsolete. From this setting the present investigation developed.

[11] Cairns, Laura, *A Scientific Basis for Health Instruction in Public Schools*, pp. 417-418.

CHAPTER II
The Investigation

STATEMENT AND DEFINITION OF THE PROBLEM

THE PROBLEM which confronted the investigator in this study may be concisely stated: Can the study of the relation of food to physical well-being in high school biology classes be truly educative? He will attempt to solve this problem by determining whether or not the outcomes of instruction are of such a nature that they function in the daily lives of the boys and girls. If in some instances the outcomes are significant, and in other instances they are not significant, then the writer will attempt to interpret the conditions in the experimental situations which may account for the variation in the results obtained.

The outcomes of instruction are so diversified in nature that the investigator cannot hope to study all of them, but, rather, must resort to the selection of a few for intensive study and rely on the more descriptive means of evaluation for evidence of other outcomes not studied so intensively.

It appears that any truly educative experience should result in the increased use of knowledge as a basis for intelligent action. To attack the problem from this angle means that one must have an objective measure of newly acquired knowledge, else he cannot be sure that observed changes are related to increased understanding. Then it is necessary to select situations in which to study the use pupils make of knowledge acquired.

Two such situations were selected for intensive study in this experimental investigation: the first is the attitude shown by pupils toward the selection of their daily diets; the second is their application of principles to the interpretation of current food advertisements. Descriptive means of appraisal were selected as appropriate to determine whether or not boys and girls demonstrate interest, enthusiasm, initiative, and understandings in the experimental learning situations comparable to those demonstrated when studying the more usual curriculum materials.

The problem of this study is related to other problems which face the curriculum maker: Should the study of nutrition in high school be limited to those who take home economics? Is the study of those basic principles which underlie the selection of one's diet of interest and importance for boys and girls alike? Psychologists tell us that during adolescence boys and girls are prone to experiment widely. How are we to prevent these adolescents from experimenting in a detrimental fashion with their own diet when the negative results of such experimentation are not forthcoming until months or years after the experiments? How can health be taught? Should it be taught in a separate course, or should it permeate the entire school curriculum? Should it be taught in courses taken by the majority of pupils or only in elective courses? Is a laboratory essential in the teaching of those matters of health that have to do with the relation of food to physical well-being? These are but a few of the many related problems on which this study may shed some light.

It seems essential to accept certain basic considerations in order to undertake this experiment.

1. High school biology courses as commonly given contribute relatively little to the understanding and use of those principles which have to do with the relation of food to health.
2. If experiences related to health are acceptable and profitable to the pupil, they belong in the curriculum because of their social worth.
3. Adolescent boys and girls in general are not using understandings concerning the relation of food to their own well-being to an extent desirable in terms of their health.
4. An enlarged understanding of the generalizations concerning health can profitably be achieved at the secondary school level.

STEPS IN PROCEDURE

This outline shows in concise form the procedure followed by the investigator.

1. The selection and organization of the teaching materials.
2. The construction of suitable instruments for use in measuring the results of instruction.

3. The selection of experimental situations—
   a. To study changes and the persistence of those changes.
   b. To study changes obtained by different teachers in various other situations.
   c. To determine the proportion of the changes due to practice effect on the pretests.
4. The provision of means of securing descriptive examples of pupil behavior.
5. The analysis of the results of the tests—
   a. To determine the changes, the significance of the changes, and the proportion of the changes that can be attributed to the experimental factor.
   b. To make sure that the tests used are measuring different factors.
   c. To find whether or not the pupils improve in their ability to integrate the factors measured.

Step one, the selection and organization of the teaching materials, is treated in Chapter III. Step two, the construction of the measuring instruments is given in Chapter IV. Steps four and five are included in Chapter V. Step three, dealing with the experimental situations, follows in this chapter.

DESCRIPTION OF THE EXPERIMENTAL SITUATIONS

The Lincoln School of Teachers College, Columbia University, the situation of the first experiment, is a private experimental school for nursery school, elementary school, and high school pupils. There are approximately three hundred boys and girls in the junior and senior high schools. The school population is rather cosmopolitan, but not representative because of selective factors of tuition and ability.

Plans for conducting the experiment at the Lincoln School were made during the spring of 1936. A great deal of preliminary work was necessary. Few books contained any extensive treatment of the subject in a form usable by this age group. Suitable illustrative materials were needed and were secured from many sources, such as government bulletins, educational materials from food manufacturers, and recent periodicals. Reference books had to be checked and supplemented with new ones which gave promise of being useful.

Experiments which could be used in the classroom were selected. A study was made of techniques for using animals effectively in the classroom. Every effort was made to be prepared to conduct the experiment in an interesting fashion.

The experimental group consisted of twenty-five ninth grade boys and girls, and twenty-five tenth grade boys and girls. Forty other ninth and tenth grade boys and girls acted as a control group by taking all the tests without participating in the rest of the experiment. All pupils were tested again a year after their study for evidence of retention.

The author was fortunate in having expert guidance and counsel throughout the experiment. One nutrition student from Teachers College mixed the diets and supervised the animal experimentation. Another advanced nutrition student was present in the classroom and contributed much to the class discussion. The school home economics teacher was associated with the class throughout the experiment. She taught the class on several occasions. Her help in preparing food exhibits and in the discussion of cooking was invaluable.

Much effort was spent to guarantee that all possible evidence concerning the effects of these experiences would be recorded. A parents' meeting was called and the proposed experiment was discussed with them with the hope that they would observe child behavior resulting from the experiences provided and would record such behavior for the investigator. Stenographic records were made of all that went on during the class periods with the thought that some questions asked, some statements made, some unique pupil-contributions might give additional evidence of the effectiveness of the instruction. Notebooks were carefully read to discover unusual contributions. Records were kept of informal conversations with pupils. Parents cooperated by sending in statements reflecting their children's interests, preferences, or concern about foods at home.

In order to increase the practical value of the investigation, it was deemed advisable to ask public school teachers in varied situations to cooperate in the study. Accordingly, the following letter was sent to biology teachers whom the investigator thought would be interested in trying out the experiment.

The unit of work which I am eager to have tried by biology and science teachers in different situations is described in the following pages. The unit deals with the relation of food to physical well-being, and the approach is one which I have found appeals to my own high school boys and girls; namely, the approach that through the application of the newer knowledge of nutrition to one's own dietary, one may have a superior and vibrant condition of health as opposed to just an ordinary one. The subject matter covered is essentially the subject matter covered in Sherman, H. C., *Food and Health,* published by The Macmillan Company, New York, with special emphasis upon the body's need and use of energy, minerals, and vitamins.

The emphasis upon the body's need for energy is achieved through work with a respiration calorimeter, through crude analyses of the energy value of foods, and through experiments with rats where the calorie intake is limited. The emphasis upon minerals is achieved through ash analysis of foods. The emphasis upon vitamins is achieved by a study of the various vitamins and their effect upon the body and through experiments with rats, pigeons, and guinea pigs, using diets deficient in one vitamin. In the study of the pupil's own dietary, Professor Rose's share values of foods have been used. This technique is the one which she has so ably described in her book *Foundations of Nutrition,* and seems an excellent device in enabling boys and girls to get a workable picture of their needs and how to meet them.

There is available much illustrative material for use in connection with these experiments and considerable good reference material. The unit takes approximately thirty class periods for completion.

I am glad to give you my experience with this array of subject matter and a description of all of the teaching devices used. You should, of course, be free to teach this material with the needs of your own pupils in mind, and according to your own best techniques.

I have developed appropriate instruments for measuring the results of instruction. These include a test of knowledge, an advertisement interpretation test which measures the pupils' ability to discern the truth in statements taken from various advertisements, and an attitudes scale which measures the pupils' attitude concerning the foods they eat.

I have tried out this material in the Lincoln School of Teachers College, and have had a most enthusiastic acceptance of it. I am confident that boys and girls in other high schools will enjoy and profit from a careful and scientific study of materials having to do with the relation of food to one's physical well-being.

I believe that most biology courses throughout our country make little contribution to the adolescent's knowledge of the relation of food to health, and I desire to secure evidence for or against this hypothesis. I hope that you can experiment with me.

A number of well-trained, experienced teachers who could adapt their programs to experimentation were finally selected to cooperate in this study. During the spring of 1937 eleven teachers tried out the organization in their classes, while the classes of two other biology teachers served as a control. The succeeding pages give a short description of each of the selected school situations.

School A. Residential suburban town near a large Eastern metropolis. One small manufacturing concern. Population 5,669. One four-year public high school, co-educational.

School B. Residential city situation in an agricultural district, near a large Eastern metropolis. Population 5,144. One four-year public high school, co-educational.

School C. The largest city of a small Southeastern state. Industrial center manufacturing steel, paper, cotton, and leather goods. Population 106,597. Spends a million dollars annually on education. One of three large public senior high schools. White population only.

School D. Middle-sized, rather isolated city in oil region of western Pennsylvania. Formerly a rather prosperous manufacturing center. Population decrease from 1920 to 1930—now 11,595. One public high school. Many children of foreign laborers.

School E. A consolidated school in a rural, agricultural region of central Pennsylvania.

School F. Large Middlewestern industrial center, automobiles and glass manufacturing, meat packing, oil refining. Population 290,718. Progressive public school system. 61,000 pupils in schools. School F is a modern high school, co-educational. Library and art museum in city.

School G. Large Eastern manufacturing center. Population 442,327. School population 99,746. 3,200 teachers. School G is one of seven large public high schools. City has fairly good library and art museum. Has a teacher of health education.

School H. Large private school in New York City. Progressive methods used. Co-educational.

School I. Small industrial city near a large Eastern metropolis. Population 21,206. School population largely foreign. One large four-year public high school, co-educational.

Approximately one thousand pupils participated in this study. Complete data have been collected on four hundred of these pupils. The time devoted to the investigation in each school depended on the amount of time given to the teaching of biology. In most schools, five hours a week for six weeks was allowed for the experiment.

Each participating teacher received the complete outline of suggested teaching materials, mimeographed copies of all tests for each pupil, scoring keys for the tests, lists of reference materials, and descriptions of proposed activities. (See Chapter III for the detailed information.) Assistance was also given each teacher in securing the laboratory animals, and reference books were purchased for schools which could not meet this expense. An expert in nutrition mixed the food for the experimental animals. The investigator visited all schools except three which were not within easy traveling distance to observe the progress of the experiment.

The experimental procedure involved the administering of initial tests of information, attitudes, and the application of principles, the teaching of the unit, and the giving of final tests. No instruction in nutrition was given to the control group.

The results in certain schools were limited by a lack of pupil reference material beyond the described minimum, and in two situations by a set course of study in science which somewhat lessened the time allotted to the experiment. One group did not make the respiration apparatus, the use of which was considered a valuable experience for the pupils. In this same school no laboratory animals were used. Some of the schools had such poorly equipped laboratories that only a few of the experiments could be done.

In contrast to the above limitations the teacher in School B added his own creative effort to the suggestions given, thus enriching the classroom experiences with varied reference material and with interesting supplementary activities and tests.

The organization of the educational experiences for use in teaching nutrition in biology classes follows in the succeeding chapter.

CHAPTER III

Organization of the Educational Experiences

STEP ONE

THE FIRST STEP in the development of the materials of instruction was to study and define the needs of adolescents for functional understandings in regard to nutrition. These needs have been discussed in the Introduction. It is important, however, to review them at this time. Health is dependent upon good nutrition; a prolonged lack of any essential food nutrient results in widespread disturbance of function and often of structure; optimal health for any individual is dependent upon the best combination of all essential food nutrients in his diet. Recent developments in the field of nutrition are of such importance that they offer abundant rewards in human welfare. The shift from rural to urban life has made man more dependent on others to produce his foods. Essential food nutrients are removed in some refining processes. The variety of available foods from which one selects his daily fare has increased manifold. Customs, advertisements, whims, and taste are not in any sense adequate guides for adolescents to follow in the selection of diet. The treatment of nutrition in biology textbooks gives little help. Adolescents are vitally concerned with any factor which they realize affects their rapidly maturing bodies. Their questions in this area show their keen interest and they tend to experiment widely, rejecting customary behaviors and substituting new ones. The results of experiments in diet are apt to be so delayed that harmful diet habits become established. The rapid physiological changes which occur in this period, with the accompanying mental, emotional, and social implications, call for a vital type of education for healthful and wholesome living.

STEP TWO

The second step in the development of the materials of instruction was to define the area in terms of outcomes. These outcomes were expressed as declarative sentences summarizing the understandings which are important for the lay public. They represent a digest of fundamental nutritional truths expressed in recent authoritative books on nutrition and physiology, and selected in terms of the needs and interests of adolescents, possible social usefulness, and their appropriateness for use in biology classes.

Major Generalization and Contributory Ideas

Food intake is closely related to physical well-being. A prolonged lack of any essential food nutrient results in widespread disturbance of function and often of structure. Starting with a normal body, an intake of each essential food nutrient, which just meets requirements, results in passable health; an optimal intake of each essential food nutrient results in physical vigor.

1. The body needs foods to supply energy and an optimal supply of these foods is close to minimal need:
   a. The body needs energy every moment for muscle tonus and other vital processes:
      (1) When at rest, energy is spent in maintaining circulation, respiration, and other internal processes as well as in maintaining muscular tone.
      (2) Activity, age, and size influence the energy needs of the body.
      (3) The amount of energy needed by the body is measured in terms of calories:
         (*a*) Basal energy metabolism is the rate of expenditure of energy by a person who is awake, relaxed, lying still, and who has not eaten any food during the preceding twelve hours. It is about 70 calories per hour for the average man of 70 kilograms (154 lbs.) weight.
         (*b*) The average adult spends about 100 calories per hour just sitting still; about 2,500 calories per day if engaged in light work.
      (4) The body derives energy from carbohydrates, fats, and proteins.
         (*a*) Carbohydrates may be used for energy as glucose, stored temporarily as glycogen, or converted into body fat.
         (*b*) Fats may be used for energy or stored as body fat.
         (*c*) Proteins are used in building and repairing body tissues; parts may be used for energy or stored as body fat.

   b. Intake of energy-producing foods should be only slightly above minimal need:
      (1) A superfluity of food leads to indigestion, to fatness, or to both.
         (*a*) An oversupply of energy-producing foods may limit one's intake of other essential nutrients.

(*b*) With normal metabolism, body fat originates as surplus fuel.

(2) Too meager food intake depletes the body of its normal stores of fat:

(*a*) Underweight people become easily fatigued.

(*b*) Underweight people have depleted reserves in time of need.

2. The body needs foods for growth, repair, and reproduction; an optimal supply of these body-building foods is considerably above minimal need.

a. Proteins which yield the correct amino acids are necessary for all normal cellular growth, and an optimal supply of these is about 50 per cent over minimal need.

b. Minerals are necessary for all normal cellular growth, particularly for skeletal growth; they serve a regulative function; an optimal supply of those needed in largest amounts (calcium, phosphorus, and iron) is from 100 to 300 per cent over minimal needs.

3. The body needs regulative and protective foods; an optimal supply of some of these is several times greater than minimal need:

a. Vitamin A, fat-soluble, found in fish oil, milk, and eggs or its precursor carotene, found in yellow vegetables, is needed by the body throughout its entire life cycle; an optimal intake is at least four times as great as minimal need.

b. Vitamin B, water-soluble, found in fruits, vegetables, milk, eggs, and whole grains, is needed by the body for normal food selection and usage; an optimal intake is several times a minimal intake.

c. Vitamin C, ascorbic acid, water-soluble, easily destroyed by heat, found in fruits, vegetables, and milk, is needed by the body for normal nutrition; an optimal intake is at least twice and probably several times that of minimal need.

d. Vitamin D, fat-soluble, sometimes called the sunshine vitamin or the antirachitic vitamin, found in fish oils, egg yolk, and milk, is needed by the body for normal use of calcium and phosphorus; an optimal intake is several times that of minimal need.

e. Vitamin G, water-soluble, found in eggs, liver, lean meats, vegetables, and fruits, is essential to growth, nutrition, and vitality at all ages; an optimal intake is at least four times that of minimal need.

f. Vitamin E, the anti-sterility vitamin, is widely distributed in foods, and a diet adequate in other respects will furnish enough of this vitamin.

g. New discoveries concerning these protective and regulatory foods are tending to differentiate other vitamins and to disclose their value as foods.

4. Each cell within the body must have a continual supply of food and

oxygen for its vital processes; waste materials resulting from these processes must be removed from the body.

a. Foods are prepared for distribution and use by digestion.
- (1) Digestion takes place in a food tube known as the alimentary canal.
  - (*a*) The canal consists of mouth cavity, throat cavity, gullet, stomach, small intestine, and large intestine.
  - (*b*) Insoluble food particles are made diffusible by enzymes found in the digestive juices.
  - (*c*) The salivary glands of the mouth cavity secrete saliva, an alkaline fluid containing the enzyme ptyalin, which changes starch to sugar.
  - (*d*) The gastric glands of the stomach secrete the gastric juice, an acid fluid containing the enzymes rennin, which curdles milk, and pepsin, which splits proteins.
  - (*e*) Digestion is completed in the intestine.
    - *a′* The bile from the liver makes the food alkaline, greatly facilitating the action of other digestive juices.
    - *b′* The pancreatic juice from the pancreas contains a starch-digesting enzyme, a fat-digesting enzyme, and a protein-digesting enzyme.
    - *c′* The intestinal juice from the intestinal glands contains a starch-digesting enzyme, a protein-digesting enzyme, and sugar-digesting enzymes.
  - (*f*) The digested food diffuses through the intestinal wall into the blood stream.
    - *a′* Digested carbohydrates and proteins pass through the intestinal wall into the blood stream, digested fats into the lacteals and thence into the blood stream.
    - *b′* Undigested portions, refuse, pass through the large intestine and are removed from the body.

b. Energy is released from food by oxidation within each body cell.
- (1) Vital processes are continually going on in the cells.
- (2) Food serves as the source of materials and energy for these processes.
- (3) Oxygen liberates energy from food by oxidation within the cells.
- (4) Cells use energy from oxidation for all these vital processes.
- (5) Waste products are continually produced by cells.

c. The lymph bathes the cells of the body, allowing the passage of materials to and from them.

d. The blood distributes to all parts of the body materials needed by cells and collects wastes given off by cells from all parts of the body.
- (1) The liquid portion of the blood plasma contains about 90 per

cent water, 8 per cent proteins and amino acids, slightly less than 2 per cent fats, sugars, and mineral matter, and traces of hormones and vitamins.

(2) Red corpuscles and white corpuscles float in the blood plasma; red corpuscles carry oxygen and white corpuscles combat disease germs.

(*a*) When oxygen is plentiful, as in the lungs, the hemoglobin of the red blood corpuscles combines with it forming oxy-hemoglobin.

(*b*) When oxygen is limited, the oxy-hemoglobin liberates oxygen, again forming hemoglobin.

(3) The blood circulates in a closed circulatory system. This system includes a four-chambered heart, arteries, capillaries, and veins.

(4) The blood passes from the left ventricle into the aorta, into arteries leading to all parts of the body, into capillaries in all parts of the body, into veins leading back to the heart, into the right auricle, into the right ventricle, into the pulmonary artery, into the pulmonary capillaries, into pulmonary veins, into the left auricle and thence again into the left ventricle.

(5) The blood from the capillaries of the small intestine flows through the portal vein to the liver where it again flows through capillaries before going back to the heart.

e. The blood and lymph are relatively stable in composition, concentration, and temperature.

(1) The blood gains sugar from the glycogen of the liver and loses it to the body cells.

(2) The blood gains sugar, fat, amino acids, mineral matter, and vitamins from the digestive tract and loses them to cells throughout the body.

(3) The blood gains water from the digestive tract and from the cells of the body through oxidation of food and loses it through the kidneys, sweat glands, and lungs.

(4) The blood gains oxygen from the lungs and loses it to the body cells.

(5) The blood gains carbon dioxide from the body cells and loses it through the lungs.

(6) The blood gains nitrogenous wastes from the body cells and loses it through the kidneys.

(7) The blood gains heat from oxidation in the cells of the body and loses it from the lungs and body surface.

5. Mankind has lived through the ages on "whole foods" as contrasted with the highly refined foods used today.

6. Foods may be classed according to the essentials they furnish, which in turn serve as a basis for selection of a widely varying optimal diet:

a. Breadstuffs and other grain products are economical sources of energy and proteins but not of minerals and vitamins.
   (1) Most of the mineral and vitamin content of grains is in the outer coat or bran, and in the embryo or germ.
   (2) The nutritive value of all grain or cereal products can be greatly increased by using them in the whole grain form.

b. Sugars make their sole contribution as sources of energy.

c. Fats are chiefly significant as sources of energy; some are also important as sources of vitamins A and D.

d. Muscle meats, including fish and poultry, are rich in protein or fat or both, but show about the same mineral deficiencies and vitamin deficiencies as breadstuffs.

e. Fruits and vegetables are very important as sources of mineral elements and vitamins.

f. Milk is the most efficient of all foods for use in making good the deficiencies of the grains in supplying an optimal diet.

g. Eggs rank high as sources of phosphorus, iron, and vitamins.

h. A higher level of health through improved nutrition may be attained by careful selection of foods:
   (1) Take at least half the total food calories in the form of protective foods—milk and its products, fruits, vegetables, and eggs; take breadstuffs and cereal products largely in the "whole grain" form.
   (2) Spend as much for milk and its products, and as much for fruits and vegetables, as is spent for meats, including fish and poultry.

7. The newer knowledge of nutrition indicates that, starting with a normal body, optimal nutrition results in physical vigor:
   a. It increases the quality of daily health and vigor, including resistance to disease.
   b. It enables one better to preserve the characteristics of youth.
   c. Barring accidents, it prolongs the prime of life, fostering early maturity and postponing senility.
   d. Barring accidents, it prolongs the total life span.

STEP THREE

The third step was to explore the major aspects of man's experience, as then outlined by the Committee on the Function of Science in General Education of the Progressive Education Association, to make sure that the generalizations as stated have an expressible direct relation to these major life experiences. Some of these are expressed as questions. These implications are listed in the following manner to help teachers see the kinds of applications which closely relate these nutrition experiences to the daily lives of the pupils.

Some Implications of the Proposed Materials Related to the Major Aspects of Man's Experience

Human Development

1. What are the relationships between optimal diet and physiological growth?
2. What effect has optimal diet on maturation? On length of life? On postponing senility?
3. What effect has optimal diet on the future of the race?
4. To what extent shall one rely upon one's appetite?

Maintenance of Personal and Public Health

1. What degenerative diseases come as a result of diet deficiencies?
2. What relationship exists between bodily vigor and resistance to certain infectious disease? Between bodily vigor and recovery from such disease?
3. What weaknesses does a body possess when it does not have sufficient of these protective foods?
4. What is the result in quality of life of having an abundance of the protective foods as well as all of the other essentials in optimal amounts?
5. What are the consequences of applying intelligence to the selection, preparation, and use of food?
6. What are the consequences one may expect from placing a blind faith in the demands of one's appetite?
7. How do these implications affect one's attitude toward institutional life?
8. How are these relationships between diet and health likely to change one's relations to hospitals, to research institutions, to clinics, to school health, to absences from school, to the work of boards of health, etc.?
9. What are the relationships to the expenditure of public moneys for public health?

Home and Family Life

1. What significance would these nutrition understandings have in the allotment of money for the purchase of food?
2. How would these nutrition understandings probably affect one's daily diet?
3. What would be their effect upon the family's attitudes toward illness?
4. What are possible relationships to success and happiness?
5. What are possible relationships to economic security?

6. What are possible relationships to quality of family life?
7. What are probable relationships to the care of expectant mothers?
8. What are probable relationships of bearing children to nutritional status of mother?
9. What are probable relationships to infant health and care?
10. What are probable relationships to infant morbidity and mortality?
11. What are probable relationships to care of the aged?

Social-Civic Life

1. How would nutrition understandings affect one's leadership in all kinds of community projects?
2. How would they affect the work of the church organizations for the welfare of others?
3. How would they tend to affect the kinds of meals served at dinners?
4. What is the bearing of nutrition knowledge on the sale of candy, etc., for purposes of raising money for various activities?
5. What customs might be modified?
6. How shall one be more intelligent in regard to charity?
7. Shall money, or food, be given to the poor? If food, what food, etc?

Economic-Industrial Life

1. What would be the effect of such knowledges and actions on the consumption of foods?
2. What would be the possible changes in advertising and marketing of foodstuffs?
3. What changes in the products offered on the market might result from such widespread knowledge?
4. What effect would such general practices have upon the standards of processing and marketing foods?
5. What changes in the food crops raised might be brought about?

Previously Known Generalizations

1. What is the possible relationship between diet customs and the success of some forms of life and the extinction of others?
2. What is the possible relationship between diet customs and the evolution of the present races of men from prehistoric times?
3. What is the possible relationship between some of the diet peculiarities of different races and the survival of those races?
4. What is the possible relationship of food customs to development of stature of various races?
5. What is the possible relationship of food customs to intellectual development?

Man's Thinking about Life and the Universe

1. What viewpoint is here suggested with regard to such matters as nationalism or internationalism?
2. How does this relate to one's attitude toward war?

3. What tie-up is suggested between these understandings and birth control?
4. What modifications should man make in his social philosophy to provide for his betterment?

STEP FOUR

It seemed important when setting up the extended experiment to write concise, definite suggestions for teachers to use in planning the organization and teaching of nutrition in their biology classes. The suggestions which follow were sent to the participating teachers early, so that they might better plan their class experiences. They are included at this time to give the reader an overview of the class procedures.

General Teaching Suggestions

The following pages define the scope of the unit on the Relation of Food to Physical Well-Being. They are not written to determine arbitrarily the subject matter included, the emphasis given, the sequence followed, or the time allotted. They are written to serve as a flexible, usable guide in selecting the approaches and activities. The author found in working with three different classes during the past year that the activities here included have teaching value, and that the time suggested is adequate for most boys and girls to grasp the essential ideas.

Six weeks is not long enough to include all the activities suggested. The teacher should feel free to modify the time allotment, to select the activities most appropriate for the local situation, to substitute other activities for those suggested here.

Many of the activities suggested are needed to enable the pupils to come to scientific understandings based upon experiences meaningful to them. Animal experimentation is fundamental in this respect. Only by participation in experiments of this kind can boys and girls really appreciate the painstaking and carefully controlled experimentation which has yielded our present knowledge of nutrition. The experiments suggested on the demonstration diet sheet yield excellent results and serve as examples of two different methods used in conducting controlled experiments. Other experiments and other diets may be substituted for those suggested. The important thing is that boys and girls live through an experiment, seeing the animals periodically, observing the effects, and recording the results in a way that allows them to compare the effects of the deficient diets with those of the control diet.

Similarly, talking about calories expended without any objective measurements is futile. Crude apparatus may be used. It is not necessary to take into consideration room temperature, barometric pressure, and relative humidity. It is important, however, that the boys and girls understand how energy expenditure can be measured, and what factors determine one's energy requirement. Several measurements with some type of apparatus should be made. These may be supplemented by descriptions of a basal metabolism apparatus, respiration calorimeter, water calorimeter, an ice calorimeter, a Douglas bag, or a bicycle ergometer. Some pupils might visit a hospital or a research laboratory.

It is interesting to measure the calories of heat given off by a guinea pig or rat in an ice calorimeter. A coffee can equipped with a rubber stopper and a glass tube to allow for breathing will serve as a container for the animal. This may be packed in a larger can well insulated from the outside. The difference in the number of grams of ice melted in four minutes when the can is empty and when the guinea pig is in it serves as a basis for calculating the number of calories given off by the animal.

Boys and girls can gain some understanding of the energy value of foods by burning a small amount of starch, fat, and protein, seeing that each yields energy, and that fat yields relatively more than the others. They can determine the moisture content of several foods by taking a hundred-calorie portion of each and drying it over the radiator. The loss in weight gives the water content. Cornstarch and lettuce give striking contrast. These dry foods may then be burned until only ash is left. The amount of organic matter and mineral matter can then be determined. Also splitting starch into carbon and water by heating in a test tube gives a basis for considering the chemical nature. Some comprehension of chemical change is essential to the understanding of the various ways of measuring energy expenditure; that is, oxygen consumed, heat given off, and carbon dioxide given off.

The process of digestion can be illustrated by this experiment: Place a dilute suspension of starch in four test tubes, add malt diastase to three of them and mix thoroughly. Add iodine to test tube having starch only and note blue color. At intervals of two minutes add iodine to other three test tubes. The starch should be completely changed to sugar in one of the tubes. The results may be further checked by testing the tubes for sugar, using Benedict's solution or Fehling's solution.

The ability of living things to oxidize sugar can be demonstrated by placing yeast, warm water, and sugar in a gas collecting bottle. This can be inverted in a water bath. The gas collected can be shown to be carbon dioxide by testing with limewater.

Dissection of a small animal aids in the study of the digestive and circulatory systems. A sheep's heart or pig's heart can be dissected to advantage also.

Food exhibits and share graphs prove useful in learning the contributions which various types of foods make to one's dietary.

The bulletin board is valuable in displaying the illustrative material, charts, and graphs that are available.

The pupils will probably wish to include many of the following in their notebooks:

Class notes on experiments, reports, etc.
Explanation of use and care of rats.
Diets fed to animals.
Graphs showing growth of animals in each cage.
Description of effects of diets on animals.
Diagram and explanation of respiration apparatus.
Table of results from tests with respiration apparatus.
Definition of calorie, metabolism, basal metabolism, digestion, respiration, share, etc.
Classification of foods according to composition.
Description of other ways of measuring energy needs of body.
Factors that affect one's energy need.
Diagram and explanation of ice calorimeter experiment.
Analysis and graph of energy expenditure.
Graph of total shares needed daily.
Graph of shares furnished by representatives of each class of foods.
Description and table of results obtained from class analyses of foods.
Description and diagram of bomb calorimeter.
Table showing function of each part of digestive system.
Description of digestion experiment.
Diagram of human circulatory system.
Description tracing course of blood through the body.
Factors affecting the stability of the blood and lymph.
Summary of present knowledge of each vitamin.
Ways of providing a safe diet.
An analysis of one's own diet.

The class might like to undertake some culminating activity, such as a food exhibit showing shares furnished by each, or an assembly program, or an exhibit and social hour for parents.

The outline entitled "Suggested Organization for Class Periods" (see p. 26) allots time about as indicated in the following table:

Pretests	2	periods
Overview	½	
Animal experimentation	3½	
Energy needs of body	6	
Energy value of food	2	
Body-building materials	2	
Body function	4½	
Regulating foods	3½	
Selecting safe diet	3	
Review	1	
Final tests	2	
Total	30	periods

The suggested questions, problems, and topics for each of these class periods are as follows:

Period 1—Pretests.
Period 2—Pretests.
Period 3—Overview of unit.
Period 4—How can we demonstrate some of the essentials of a good diet? (Animal experimentation)
Period 5—What are the energy needs of the body?
Period 6—In what ways can we determine the energy needs of the body?
Period 7—How can we measure the energy needs of the body with the portable respiration apparatus?
Period 8—*a.* What is the condition of the animals on the various diets?
b. What is basal metabolism?
Period 9—What factors influence basal metabolism?
Period 10—What is the energy cost of activity?
Period 11—How can one calculate and show graphically one's total daily energy requirement?
Period 12—How can we measure the energy needs of a small animal by means of a home-made ice calorimeter?
Period 13—*a.* What is the condition of the animals on the various diets?
b. Why are some foods richer in energy than others?
Period 14—*a.* How can we measure the energy value of foods?
b. How could an extensive use of fats, sugars, and starches affect one's dietary?
Period 15—What body-building foods are essential?
Period 16—How are foods digested?
Period 17—How are digested foods absorbed into the body?
Period 18—*a.* What is the condition of the animals on the various diets?
b. How is energy liberated from foods within the body?
Period 19—How are foods distributed within the body?
Period 20—How are the blood and lymph kept in a stable condition?
Period 21—What regulative foods are needed by the body?
Period 22—Vitamins A and D.
Period 23—*a.* What is the condition of the animals on the various diets?
b. Vitamins B and G.
Period 24—*a.* Vitamin C.
b. Summary of the vitamins.
Period 25—Ways of providing a safe diet.
Period 26—Analysis of own daily diet.
Period 27—Analysis of own daily diet and comparison with standard.
Period 28—*a.* What is the condition of the animals on the various diets?
b. Exhibit of foods rich in each dietary essential which one needs to consider when selecting one's diet.
Period 29—Final test.
Period 30—Final test.

STEP FIVE

The fifth step was to select appropriate problems with activities useful in their solution, and to arrange these problems in a tentative workable schedule for use as an approximate guide for time allotment and sequence. Every effort was made to include as wide a variety of suitable experiences as possible for the solution of each problem so that pupils and teachers would have an opportunity to select those activities which interested them most. Every effort was made to have the problems, activities, and assignments of interest to adolescents. Teachers were urged to vary the assignments and activities in terms of the interests of their pupils.

Suggested Organization for Class Periods

Period 1

Activities: Pretests.
Assignment:

1. Keep a complete record of everything you eat for one day. List under four headings; namely, Breakfast, Lunch, Dinner, and Between Meals. Indicate amounts as nearly as possible.

Period 2

Activities: Pretests.
Assignment:

1. Keep a careful notebook. Include class notes, record of feeding experiments, record of class experiments, illustrative materials in magazines and newspapers. Bring them for bulletin board.

Period 3

Questions and Problems:

1. Why should we study about the foods we eat?
   a. What relationship exists between diet and health?
   b. Are we enjoying vigorous, buoyant health, or merely passable health?
   c. What has food to do with our condition?
   d. What are the important things to be considered in the study of the relation of food to our physical condition?

Activities:

1. Overview of Unit:
   a. Read and discuss selected portions of *Food and Health,*[1] Chapter XIX, or,

[1] For authors, publishers, etc., see reference bibliography on pages 54 to 56.

b. Read and discuss portions of pamphlet, *Nutritional Improvement in Health and Longevity,* or,
c. Have class discussion around important problems, or,
d. Give an overview in exposition form.

References:
1. *Food and Health,* Chap. XIX, "The Option Which Our Present Knowledge Offers"; Chap. I, "The Importance of an Intelligent Use of Food"; Chap. II, "Avoidance of Injury and Exploitation."
2. *Nutritional Improvement in Health and Longevity.*

Assignment:
1. Find out all you can about the use of animals in testing foods. Be ready to tell any experience in feeding pets or farm animals that might aid the class in determining the needs of our bodies.

PERIOD 4

Questions and Problems:
1. How can we demonstrate some of the essentials of a good diet?
    a. Why are white rats so suitable for carrying out experiments with diets?
    b. What other animals are also suitable for diet experiments and for what experiments should we prefer them?
    c. How can we set up feeding experiments to be sure that we are measuring the thing which we wish to find out about?
    d. How should we prepare the diets for these experiments?
    e. How can we best observe and study the experiments undertaken?

Activities:
1. Acquaint everyone with feeding experiments. Discuss and record diets fed each cage, and what each factor contributes to diet. Discuss methods of selecting animals, rate of growth, life history, and usableness for specific experimental purposes. Pass some animals around the class in large jar. Everyone begin graph on growth of rats. Use Nutrition charts (see p. 55)—"Growth as an Index of Nutrition" and "Growth May Be Controlled by Diet."
2. Extract all vitamins from a small amount of meat as suggested for making meat residue for feeding experiments.

References:
1. *Teaching Nutrition to Boys and Girls,* pp. 157-190—"The White Rat and Feeding Experiments."
2. *Laboratory Experiments in Nutrition* (Booklet).

Assignment:

Find out all you can about the energy needs of the body.
Be ready to discuss them in class.

PERIOD 5

Questions and Problems:

1. What are the energy needs of the body?
   a. For what purposes does the body always spend energy?
   b. What factors influence the amounts of energy which the body spends?
   c. How does the body get its energy?
   d. How does this energy-getting process compare with the oxidation of fuels outside the body?
   e. Why do people get fat? Thin?
   f. Should our body weight fluctuate widely or show a rather uniform increase until we reach maturity?
   g. Can we trust our appetites to tell us when we have eaten enough? Why or why not?

Activities

1. Illustrate kinds of food, starch, sugar, fat and protein; burn small portions of each to show that they liberate energy.
2. Determine what foods are made of by heating a small portion in a test tube and splitting:
   a. Starch, sugar, and fat into water and carbon.
   b. Protein into water and carbon and noting foul odors characteristic of all proteins.
3. Discuss energy needs of the body.

References:

1. *Food and Health,* Chap. III—"Energy for Our Daily Work"; Chap. IV—"Foods as Fuels for the Energy Needs of the Body"; Chap. V—"The Control of Body Weight"; Chap. VI—"The Energy Needs in Childhood and with Advancing Age."
2. *Teaching Nutrition to Boys and Girls,* pp. 1-25—"Foods Make a Difference."
3. *Foundations of Nutrition,* Chap. III—"The Energy Requirements of Adults."
4. *Birds as Heat Engines* (Bulletin).
5. *Reptiles Used in Study of Human Physiology* (Bulletin).

Assignment:

Find out how we can measure the body's need for energy.

PERIOD 6

Questions and Problems:

1. In what ways can we determine the energy needs of the body?
   a. If a person's weight does not change over a period of time, can we say that his food intake is just sufficient to meet his energy demands?

b. How can we measure the heat given off by the body with a respiration chamber? A water calorimeter? An ice calorimeter?

c. What is a calorie?

d. How can we determine the energy needs of the body by measuring the products of the oxidation of food within the body in terms of carbon dioxide given off? In terms of oxygen consumed?

Activities:

1. Define and illustrate the calorie. Show a liter of water; show a cube ten centimeters on a side; show the relation between a liter and a kilogram for water. Heat a known quantity of water a few degrees and calculate the calories required.
2. Compare Centigrade and Fahrenheit thermometers.
3. Visualize calorie in English system. One quart of water is somewhat less than one liter of water. Two degrees Fahrenheit are somewhat more than one degree Centigrade. A calorie is roughly the amount of heat necessary to raise the temperature of a quart of water two degrees Fahrenheit.
4. Have a few members of the class determine the amount of energy they are expending in terms of the amount of carbon dioxide they are exhaling. To do this, have each exhale for five minutes through a large jar of limewater. After the calcium carbonate has settled in the jar, decant the clear liquid. Transfer the remainder to a small beaker. Allow it to dry over the radiator. Weigh the residue. With an average respiration quotient, 0.82, each gram of calcium carbonate formed represents the liberation of 1.32 calories within the body.

References:

1. *Biology and Human Welfare,* pp. 194-195—"What Calories Are."
2. *Foundations of Nutrition,* pp. 11-25.
3. *Energy Consumption in Physical and Mental Effort* (Bulletin).

Assignment:

Find out about the measurement of energy expenditure in one way in detail. Perhaps some member of the class will construct an ice calorimeter for use in class later. Some pupil might visit a hospital and find out how basal metabolism is measured.

PERIOD 7

Questions and Problems:

1. How can we measure the body's need for energy with the portable respiration apparatus?

   a. What gas is in the can of the apparatus?

   b. How does this gas circulate when tests are taken?

   c. What chemical is in the can? Why is it there?

   d. What gas does the subject remove from the circulating air?

   e. What products does the subject add to the circulating air?

f. How can the calories produced by the subject be determined from these measurements?

Activities:

1. Demonstrate the construction and operation of the respiration apparatus. Run a demonstration test. Calculate daily energy expenditure of patient. Each cubic centimeter of oxygen consumed corresponds to 0.004825 calories expended by the subject.
2. Run additional tests and calculate daily expenditure of energy.

References:

Same as for Period 6.

Assignment

1. Make cross sectional diagram of the respiration apparatus in your notebook and explain its operation.
2. Keep a careful record of tests and calculations performed.
3. Do further reading in references given for Periods 5 and 6.

PERIOD 8

Questions and Problems:

1. What is the condition of the animals on the various diets?
   a. Do they show any differences in any respect?
   b. Have they grown equally well?
2. Basal metabolism:
   a. Define it.
   b. Why is it taken in a reclining position?
   c. Why is it taken 12 to 14 hours after meals?
   d. Why not take it when the patient is asleep?
   e. What factors cause the greatest variation in basal metabolism?

Activities:

1. Handle animals in front of class and discuss condition.
2. Pass one or more animals around class for inspection. (Make sure that there is no possibility of mixing them.)
3. Discuss growth and have pupils plot it on their growth chart.
4. Discuss basal metabolism, factors that influence it, and standards for calculating it.

References:

1. *Foundations of Nutrition,* pp. 42-46—"The Basal Metabolism." Also see basal metabolism for factors in index.

Assignment:

1. Make entries on growth charts.
2. Determine your own basal energy needs in terms of age, weight, and sex.
3. Determine your own basal energy needs in terms of age, body surface, and sex.

PERIOD 9

Questions and Problems:

1. What factors influence basal metabolism?
   - *a.* How does it vary with age?
   - *b.* How does it vary with size?
   - *c.* How does it vary with sex?
   - *d.* What other factors affect it?

Activities:

1. Discuss factors influencing basal metabolism, and basal energy needs calculated by members of the class.
2. Run several more tests with respiration apparatus. Try if possible to secure some evidence for some of the above variables.

References:

Same as for Period 8.

Assignment:

1. Complete calculations in notebooks on tests run in class.
2. Find out about the energy cost of activities. Secure any evidence possible, such as food consumption in different occupations, or energy cost of athletics.

PERIOD 10

Questions and Problems:

1. What is the energy cost of activities?
   - *a.* What physiological changes does one notice when spending energy rapidly? How are circulation, breathing, heat production, thirst, appetite, etc., affected?
   - *b.* How can the energy cost of activities be determined?

Activities:

1. Discuss the energy cost of activities.
2. Take pulse and breathing rate of class member before and after exercise.
3. Run several tests with respiration apparatus, first without activity, then with subject raising and lowering arms with a kilogram weight in each hand during the test.
4. Calculate the energy cost of the activity in tests made.

References:

1. *Foundations of Nutrition*, pp. 56-63—"Allowances for the Influence of Muscular Activity."
2. *Energy Consumption in Physical and Mental Effort* (Bulletin).

Assignment:

1. Complete calculation of tests made in classroom and include in notebook.

2. Make a complete analysis of how you spend your day. This will be used in calculating your energy needs for an entire day.

PERIOD 11

Questions and Problems:

1. How can one calculate and show graphically one's total daily energy requirement?

Activities:

1. Show the class how to calculate their total energy needs.
2. Have each pupil calculate his energy need and then plot it by a bar graph.

References:

Same as for Period 10.

Assignment:

1. Complete calculation of energy cost of activities, and graph of same.

PERIOD 12

Questions and Problems:

1. How can we measure the energy expenditure of a small animal by means of a home-made ice calorimeter?
   a. How is the calorimeter constructed?
   b. How does it measure the energy expenditure of the animal?
   c. What precautions have to be taken to be sure that the ice melted was melted by the animal? (Why have a control?)
   d. How do we calculate the energy expended? (Each gram of ice melted absorbs 0.08 calories.)
   e. How does the animal's rate of energy expenditure compare with your rate of expenditure in terms of body weight?

Activities:

1. Measure expenditure of energy of small animal in a home-made ice calorimeter.

References:

1. *Foundations of Nutrition,* pp. 11-12—"Ice and Water Calorimeters."

Assignment:

1. Complete all work to date in notebooks and hand them in tomorrow.

PERIOD 13

Questions and Problems:

1. What is the condition of the animals on the various diets?
   a. Do they show differences in any respect?
   b. Have they grown equally well?
2. Why are some foods so much richer in energy than others?
   a. How does fat content affect the energy value of foods?
   b. How does moisture content affect the energy value of foods?

3. How can we show the contribution which various foods make in shares?
   a. What is a share?
   b. How can we plot shares?

Activities:

1. Observe condition of animals.
2. Exhibit 100 calorie portions of food, such as lettuce, apples, bread, butter, sugar, and eggs.
3. Weigh and place in drying oven or over radiator to dry.
4. Learn to represent contributions of foods to diet in shares.

References:

1. *Foundations of Nutrition,* Chap. XVI—"Contributions Made to the Diet by Various Types of Food Materials"; also Appendix, Table I.

Assignment:

1. Keep a record of experiment on moisture content of foods in notebook.
2. Make a share graph of each food used in the experiment.

PERIOD 14

Questions and Problems:

1. How can we measure the energy value of foods?
   a. How does a bomb calorimeter work?
   b. How does it determine the energy value of foods?
   c. How else might we determine the energy value of foods? (Oxy-calorimeter)
2. How would an extensive use of fats, sugars, and starches affect one's dietary?
   a. What shares would be supplied abundantly?
   b. What shares would be deficient?

Activities:

1. Complete determination of moisture in foods selected.
2. Burn dry foods to determine organic matter and ash content.
3. Discuss measurement of energy value of foods with bomb calorimeter and oxy-calorimeter.
4. Compare and discuss shares of foods plotted.

References:

1. *Foundations of Nutrition,* pp. 30-36—"The Measurement of Energy in Food Materials."
2. *Biology and Human Welfare,* p. 194—diagram of bomb calorimeter.

Assignment:

1. Make share models of oatmeal, eggs, cheese, oranges, and spinach.
2. Find out about the use of minerals and protein in the body.

PERIOD 15

Questions and Problems:

1. What body-building foods are essential?
   a. What functions do the protein foods serve in our bodies?
   b. What minerals does the body need and what functions do they serve in the body?
      (1) What is the place of calcium in our bodies and why consider it in balancing our diet?
      (2) What is the place of phosphorus in our bodies and why consider it in balancing our diet?
      (3) What is the place of iron in our bodies and why consider it in balancing our diet?
      (4) What other minerals are found in the body?
      (5) Which of these other minerals are sometimes deficient in the diet?

Activities:

1. Complete ash analysis of foods.
2. Write mineral composition of body on the board for use in discussion.

References:

1. *Food and Health,* Chap. VIII—"Proteins and Their Amino Acids"; Chap. IX—"The Mineral Elements in Nutrition"; Chap. X—"The Significance of Being Born Calcium Poor."
2. *Foundations of Nutrition,* Chap. VIII—"Mineral Elements and Water as Body Building Material."
3. *Teaching Nutrition to Boys and Girls,* Unit II, pp. 51-62—"Taking Milk Apart" and "The Need of Calories Plus Calcium Plus Vitamin D."
4. *Biology and Human Welfare,* pp. 192-198—"What We Should Eat and Why."
5. Use Government Nutrition Charts entitled:
   a. "Protein for Building Muscle and Tissue."
   b. "Calcium for Building Strong Bones and Teeth."
   c. "Iron for Red Blood."

Assignment:

1. Write up experiment on ash analysis of foods in notebook.
2. Find out about the digestive system and how each part functions.

PERIOD 16

Questions and Problems:

1. How are foods digested?
   a. What are the chief digestive organs?
   b. How are these organs arranged in the body?
   c. What is digestion? How is it accomplished?

d. What digestion takes place in the mouth?
e. What digestion takes place in the stomach?
f. What digestion takes place in the small intestine?
g. What happens to undigested portions of food?

Activities:

1. Do experiment on digestion of starch.
2. Dissect frog or chicken to study the digestive tract.
3. Use chart of human digestive system to compare with above.
4. Make chart on blackboard and in notebooks of the digestive organ, acid or alkaline condition, juices acting, and digestion taking place.
5. Show experiment set-up to demonstrate osmosis the following day.

References:

1. *Biology and Human Welfare,* pp. 91-112—"How Are Foods Prepared for Distribution" and "Use in the Human Body."
2. *Food and Health,* Chap. VII—"Digestion."

Assignment:

1. Learn the names of the parts of the digestive system.
2. Know what digestion takes place in each organ.

PERIOD 17

Questions and Problems:

1. How are digested foods absorbed into the body?
   a. How do they go through the intestinal wall?
   b. What happens to these foods after they get through the intestinal wall?
   c. How is it that food passes readily through the intestine into the blood stream?

Activities:

1. Demonstrate osmosis experiment set-up preceding day.
2. Demonstrate diffusion of potassium permanganate crystal in still water.
3. Demonstrate diffusion of illuminating gas through a porous cup.
4. Study slides, lantern slides, or charts of intestinal wall.
5. Examine intestinal wall of a chicken.
6. Start experiment with yeast to show oxidation of food by living things.
7. Prepare two slides of living paramecia. Seal one slide around cover glass with candle wax to shut out air. Keep both slides in a moist chamber or jar until the following day. Note effect of lack of air on paramecia.
8. Wet a bottle, shake a few iron filings in it so that they stick to sides. Turn upside down in water bath and leave until the following day. Note proportion of air that combines with iron.

References:

Same as for Period 16.

Assignment:

1. Keep a careful notebook record of class activities.
2. Find out how and where food is oxidized in the body.

PERIOD 18

Questions and Problems:

1. What is the condition of the animals on the various diets?
   a. Have they grown equally well?
   b. Do they show differences in any respect? (Note state of eyes, fur, posture, respiration, temperature of feet.)
2. How is energy liberated from foods within the body?
   a. What gas did we find the body gives off? Takes in?
   b. What are the chief gases in the air? How do heated picture wire and splints behave in each?
   c. How is our respiratory system constructed?
   d. How do we breathe?
   e. How does oxygen get into the blood stream from the lungs and carbon dioxide into the lungs from the blood stream?
   f. How does our blood carry oxygen? Carbon dioxide?
   g. How does oxygen go from the blood to the cells in all parts of the body and carbon dioxide from these cells into the blood?
   h. How do cells oxidize foods at such relatively low temperatures?

Activities:

1. Observe condition of animals.
2. Examine yeast plant experiment, test gas with limewater, observe that these plants have obtained energy from the sugar through oxidation at a relatively low temperature giving off carbon dioxide.
3. Examine experiment on composition of air. Note that bottle is about one fifth filled with water. Test portion of gas with limewater, showing gas is not carbon dioxide. Show that it will not support combustion. Identify it as nitrogen. Note that oxygen united with the iron at relatively low temperature.
4. Produce pure oxygen by heating a small portion of equal parts potassium chlorate and manganese dioxide in a test tube. Show how heated picture wire and glowing splint react in pure oxygen.
5. Secure lung and windpipe from calf, pig, sheep or chicken. Study air passages and note how they are held open by cartilage rings. Note the thin moist air sacs at the end of the branched air tubes. Inflate lungs if from freshly killed animal. Note the thin serous membrane covering surface of lung that allows movement without undue friction.
6. Demonstrate inspiration and expiration by apparatus made by connecting rubber balloon to a glass tube placed through a rubber stopper in top of bell jar and by stretching rubber dam over bottom of bell jar. Then pull down on rubber dam to illustrate inspiration and release to illustrate expiration.

7. Examine charts and slides of lungs.
8. Examine live frog or tadpole. Note moist surface of skin. Compare with moist condition of lungs. Gases pass through moist surfaces more readily than through dry surfaces.
9. Take fresh blood which has been kept away from the air and shake with air in partly filled glass bottle. Note change of color from maroon to scarlet. This may also be done by placing a little fresh blood on blotting paper and watching change of color.
10. Examine own blood under microscope for red blood corpuscles. (Sterilize needle and finger with alcohol or iodine before pricking for blood.)

References:

1. *Biology and Human Welfare,* pp. 170-187—"How Is Breathing Carried on in Man?"

Assignments:

1. Write experiments in notebook.
2. Find out about the circulation of blood in the body.

PERIOD 19

Questions and Problems:

1. How are foods and oxygen distributed within the body?
   a. What are the organs of circulation?
   b. How is each constructed?
   c. How does the heart pump the blood?
   d. How do the arteries aid in the movement of the blood?
   e. How are the veins constructed to prevent backward flow?
   f. How are the capillaries constructed so that movement of fluids between them and the lymph is facilitated?
   g. How does the lymph facilitate passage of dissolved foods and gases to and from the cells?
   h. How is surplus lymph returned to the blood stream?
   i. Trace the circulation of the blood through the body.
   j. Trace the circulation of the blood through the portal system and account for this special arrangement.

Activities:

1. Dissect the heart of a calf, sheep, or pig.
2. Observe the circulation of the blood in the web of a frog's foot under the miscroscope.
3. Diagram the circulation of the blood throughout the human body; note changes in composition in the pulmonary system; throughout the body; around the small intestine; in the liver.

References:

1. *Biology and Human Welfare,* pp. 115-129—"The Organs of Circulation"; pp. 133-137—"Hygiene of the Blood and of the Circulatory System."

Assignment:

1. Diagram the circulation of the blood throughout the body (keep in notebook).
2. Trace the circulation of the blood throughout the body (keep in notebook).
3. Prepare notebooks and hand them in at next class session.

PERIOD 20

Questions and Problems:

1. How are the blood and lymph kept in a stable condition?
   a. How is the sugar, fat, amino acid, mineral and vitamin content of the blood and lymph lowered and replenished?
   b. How is the concentration of glucose in the blood regulated?
   c. How is the fat concentration of blood lymph kept relatively constant?
   d. How do the blood and lymph gain water? Lose water?
   e. How do the blood and lymph gain oxygen? Lose oxygen?
   f. How do the blood and lymph gain carbon dioxide? Lose carbon dioxide?
   g. From what sources do the blood and lymph gain nitrogenous wastes? How are they removed from these fluids?
   h. How does the blood tend to equalize temperature throughout the body?
   i. How does the blood gain heat? Lose it?

Activities:

1. Use motion pictures to illustrate the passage of materials to and from the blood stream through the lymph.
2. Heat flask of water nearly to boiling to show that gases are dissolved in water.
3. Test blood serum for presence of salt.
4. Try chilling effect of ice on wrist or back of neck (necessary to continue for some time).
5. Demonstrate cooling by evaporation.

References:

1. *Biology and Human Welfare,* pp. 113-115—"The Composition and Uses of Blood"; pp. 129-133—"Circulation and Excretion."

Assignment:

1. Make a summary outline for notebook showing how stability of blood is maintained.
2. Find out about the regulative foods which the body needs.

PERIOD 21

Questions and Problems:

1. What regulative foods are needed by the body?

a. What kinds of regulative foods are there?
b. To what extent are the various nutritive factors interrelated within the body?
c. Is it sufficient to consider our reactions to the separate nutritional factors, or must we think of our body reactions to the combinations of foods that we eat?
d. In what ways is milk of value to us?
e. Are fruits and vegetables desirable in the diet?
f. How does our need of regulative foods differ from our need of energy producing foods?

Activities:

1. Have discussion using share graphs of milk, eggs, and several fruits and vegetables.

References:

1. *Food and Health,* Chap. XI—"Six Outstanding Concepts in Nutrition, with a General Introduction to the Vitamins."
2. *Biology and Human Welfare,* pp. 199-207 (regulative foods).
3. *Foundations of Nutrition,* Chap. XVII—"Milk"; Chap. XIX—"Vegetables and Fruits."

Assignment:

1. Make share graphs of foods rich in vitamin A. (Plan on completing share graphs to make a total of twenty during the next four days.)
2. Read about vitamins A and D.
3. Prepare special reports about vitamins A and D.

PERIOD 22

Questions and Problems:

1. Of what use is vitamin A to the body? Where do we get it and how much should we have?
   a. What happens to the body when the supply is limited?
   b. How does this vitamin appear to be related to calcium and phosphorus assimilation?
   c. How much of this vitamin is desirable? What is a vitamin A unit?
   d. To what extent is it stored in the body?
   e. What are the advantages of an optimal supply of this vitamin in the body?
   f. How can we secure this vitamin in our shares of food?
   g. When might the concentrated forms be of use to us?
2. Of what use is vitamin D to the body? Where do we get it and how can we be sure we are getting an adequate amount?
   a. What happens to the body when the supply of vitamin D is limited?
   b. How is it related to calcium and phosphorus assimilation?
   c. How much vitamin D is desirable? What is a vitamin D unit?
   d. What are the advantages of an optimal supply of this vitamin?

e. To what extent is it stored in the body?
f. Where can we secure it?
g. Of what value are concentrates of this vitamin to us?

Activities:

1. Discuss these vitamins.
2. Have special reports on illustrative material.
3. Use nutrition charts on vitamin A and vitamin D in discussion.
4. Use Wisconsin Alumni Research Foundation illustrative materials.
5. Use share graphs of foods rich in vitamin A.
6. Discuss ways of increasing vitamin D content of food (milk, etc.).

References:

1. *Food and Health,* Chap. XII—"Vitamin A and Carotene"; Chap. XV—"Vitamin D and the Prevention of Rickets."
2. *Foundations of Nutrition,* Chap. X—"Vitamin A as a Regulator of Body Processes"; Chap. XIII—"Vitamin D as a Regulator of Body Processes."
3. *Teaching Nutrition to Boys and Girls,* pp. 85-98—"Finding Vitamin A."
4. "Avitaminosis in Animals." (Chart)
5. "Suggested Lesson Plans on the Vitamins A, B, C, D, E, G." (Chart)

Period 23

Questions and Problems:

1. What is the condition of the animals on the various diets?
   a. Have they grown equally well?
   b. Do they show differences in any respect? (Note hair, eyes, posture, temperature of feet, etc.).
2. Of what use is vitamin B to the body? Where do we get it and how much of it should we have?
   a. What happens to the body when the supply is limited?
   b. How is this vitamin related to appetite and nutrition?
   c. How much of this vitamin is desirable? What is a vitamin B unit?
   d. What are the advantages of an optimal supply?
   e. To what extent is this vitamin stored in the body?
   f. How can we secure this vitamin in our shares of food?
   g. What are the concentrated sources of this vitamin?
3. Of what use is vitamin G to the body? Where do we get it and how much do we need?
   a. What happens to the body when the supply of vitamin B is limited?
   b. How is this vitamin related to nutrition?
   c. How much of this vitamin is desirable? What is a vitamin G unit?
   d. What are the advantages of an optimal supply?
   e. How can we secure vitamin G in our shares of food?
   f. To what extent can the body store this vitamin?

Activities:

1. Observe condition of animals.
2. Have class discussion using illustrative material and share graphs.
3. Have reports and discuss them.
4. Use illustrative material:
   a. Nutrition charts on vitamin B and vitamin G.
   b. Wisconsin Alumni Research Foundation Charts.

References:

1. *Food and Health,* Chap. XIII—"Vitamin B"; Chap. XVI—"Vitamin G."
2. *Foundations of Nutrition,* Chap. XI—"Vitamin B as a Regulator of Body Processes"; Chap. XV—"Vitamin G as a Regulator of Body Processes."
3. "Avitaminosis in Animals." (Chart)
4. "Suggested Lesson Plans on the Vitamins A, B, C, D, E, G." (Chart)

Assignment:

1. Complete share graphs and hand in at next class session.
2. Prepare reports and find out about vitamin C.

PERIOD 24

Questions and Problems:

1. Of what use is vitamin C to the body? Where do we get it and how much do we need?
   a. What happens to the body when the supply is limited?
   b. How is this vitamin related to calcium and phosphorus assimilation?
   c. How much of this vitamin is desirable? What is a vitamin C unit?
   d. What are the advantages of an optimal supply of vitamin C?
   e. To what extent can our bodies store this vitamin?
   f. How stable is this vitamin? How does this affect relative desirability of cooked and uncooked fruits and vegetables?
   g. How does this modify our cooking?
   h. How can we secure vitamin C in our shares of food?
   i. How can we test for this vitamin?

Activities:

1. Discuss vitamin C, using illustrative material and share graphs.
2. Have discussion on special reports.
3. Use the following illustrative material:
   a. Nutrition chart on vitamin C.
   b. Wisconsin Alumni Research Foundation Charts.
4. Perform chemical tests on vitamin C to determine relative concentration in various fruit juices:
   a. Compare cider with lemon juice.

b. Titrate citrus fruit juices when fresh and after long standing to show how easily vitamin C is destroyed.

c. Titrate fruit juice before and after boiling to show destruction by heat. (The chemical dye used for this test is sodium 2:6 dichlorobenzenone indophenol. It can be purchased from the Eastman Kodak Co., Rochester, N. Y., for approximately $1.00 per gram. Dissolve one-tenth gram in 200 c.c. of water to make titration solution. This dye is blue in neutral or alkaline solution and red in acid solution. The red color fades when reduced by vitamin C.) References on this test may be found in:

(1) *Journal of Nutrition,* Vol. 12, No. 4, Oct., 1936, article by Flora Henning.

(2) *Journal of Biological Chemistry. 103,* 6871, 1933, article by Bossey and King.

(3) *Biochemical Journal, 27,* 590, 1933, article by Birch, Harris, and Ray.

References:

1. *Food and Health,* Chap. XIV—"Vitamin C."
2. *Foundations of Nutrition,* Chap. XII—"Vitamin C as a Regulator of Body Processes."
3. *Teaching Nutrition to Boys and Girls,* pp. 122-134, "Finding Vitamin C."
4. "Avitaminosis in Animals." (Chart)
5. "Suggested Lesson Plans on the Vitamins A, B, C, D, E, G." (Chart)

Assignment:

1. For your notebook make a summary outline in table form on the vitamins. Include these headings: Soluble in; Extent Stored; Stability; Effects of Extreme Deficiency; Effects of Milk Deficiency; Optimal Intake; Rich Sources.

PERIOD 25

Questions and Problems:

1. What guides may be used to safeguard our choice of foods?
2. What support is there for considerable use of so-called whole foods?
   a. How did prehistoric man meet his dietary needs?
   b. Why are whole foods a safeguard as regards:
      (1) Vitamin supply.
      (2) Mineral supply.
      (3) Normal functioning of digestive tract.
   c. What essentials are frequently lost in the refining processes?
3. Why are milk and its products, eggs, liver, fruits, and vegetables considered protective foods? To what extent should they be included in our diet?
4. What place have fats, sugars, and starches in our dietary?

Activities:

1. Class discussion, reports, etc.

References:

1. *Food and Health,* Chap. XVII—"The Probable Existence of Other Vitamins and the Concept of a Food or a Dietary as a Whole"; Chap. VIII—"The Place of Different Foods in the Dietary."
2. *Foundations of Nutrition,* Chap. XXIV—"Needs of Elementary and High School Boys and Girls"; Chap. XVI—"Contributions to the Diet Made by Various Types of Food Materials."

Assignment:

1. Have all items up-to-date in notebooks.
2. Bring a day's dietary and shares to class for use in analysis of a day's food.

PERIODS 26 AND 27

Questions and Problems:

1. How can we calculate the shares furnished in our daily dietary?
2. How can we check on the good points and the weak points in our dietary?

Activities:

1. Determine food values in shares which the boys and girls received in their day's diet. (Calculate in form similar to mimeographed sheet entitled "Contributions of Food to the Diet in Relation to Energy Value."
2. Compare daily food intake with daily requirement in shares.
3. Discuss adequacy of diets analyzed, and ways of improving them.

References:

1. Mimeographed illustrative material.
2. *Foundations of Nutrition,* pp. 386-391—"Nutritive Values Expressed as Shares of the Day's Requirement"; Appendix Table I—"Nutritive Values of Edible Portions of Foods in Shares and Vitamin Units"; Appendix Table II—"Working Plans for Construction of Adequate Diets."
3. *Food Values of Recipes in Shares and Vitamin Units.*
4. *Laboratory Handbook for Dietetics.*
5. *Nutritional Improvement in Health and Longevity.*
6. "Diets to Fit the Family Income." U. S. D. A. Farmers Bulletin 1757.
7. "The Family Food Supply." Metropolitan Life Insurance Co. Bulletin.
8. "Three Meals a Day." Metropolitan Life Insurance Co. Bulletin.

Assignment:

1. Complete calculations on own diets.
2. Review by checking through own notebook.

PERIOD 28

Questions and Problems:

1. What is the condition of the animals on the various diets?
   a. What can we learn from the growth charts?
      (1) How did low calorie animals respond to increased food intake?
      (2) How did a lack of vitamin B affect growth?
      (3) How did a lack of vitamin C affect growth?
   b. What observable effects are caused by deficiencies of each vitamin? (Note fur, eyes, condition of joints, temperature of feet, respiratory rate, etc.).
2. What practical use can we make of our knowledge concerning the relation of food to physical well-being?

Activities:

1. Observe condition of animals and complete graphs on their growth.
2. Conduct a summary discussion.
3. Prepare food exhibit using foods and share graphs.

Assignment:

1. Hand in completed notebooks.
2. Prepare for written lesson.

PERIODS 29 AND 30. FINAL TESTS.

STEP SIX

The final step was to locate illustrative and reference material for use in teaching. This proved a difficult task as little suitable material was readily available to high school pupils. Furthermore, some of the equipment necessary for the experiments proved too costly, and hence necessitated the making of simpler home-made apparatus. It was necessary to mimeograph some data for the class and to modify, develop, and mimeograph other explanatory materials. These materials included:

Chart for Determining Surface Area of Adults from Weight and Height.

Table and graph showing Basal Energy Metabolism of Boys and Girls in Terms of Body Surface.

Table and graph showing Basal Energy Metabolism of Children.

Graph showing Average Total Daily Energy Intake of Normal Boys and Girls.

Analysis of Energy Requirement of a 16-Year-Old Boy Weighing 160 Pounds.

Graph showing the Energy Requirement in Calories of a 16-Year-Old Boy Weighing 160 Pounds.
Table giving Energy Cost of Activities.
Table giving Dietary Standards in Shares for the Construction of Adequate Diets.
Graph showing Dietary Requirements in Shares for a 16-Year-Old Boy Spending 4046 Calories Daily.
Graph showing Shares Furnished by a 100 Calorie Portion of Milk.
Table showing Contributions of Food to the Diet in Relation to Energy Value.
List of Useful Reference Books, Charts, and Bulletins.
Directions for the Construction and Use of Respiration Apparatus.
Directions for Conducting Nutrition Experiments.
Description of White Rats as Laboratory Animals.
List of Sources of Supplies with Approximate Costs.

These materials are reproduced on the following pages in the order given above. The manner in which they were used in class is described in step five above.

ILLUSTRATIVE MATERIAL USED IN STEP SIX

Chart for Determining Surface Area of Adults from Weight and Height*

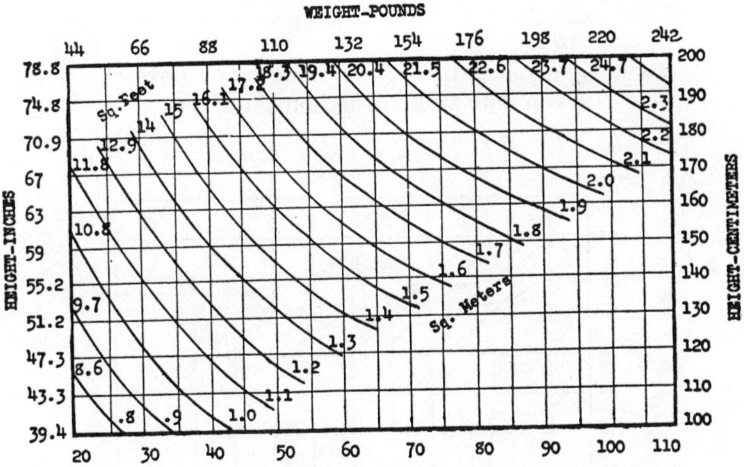

* Adapted from Rose, Mary Swartz, *Foundations of Nutrition*, p. 612. By permission of The Macmillan Company, publishers.

Basal Energy Metabolism of Boys and Girls in Terms of Body Surface*

Age in Years	Calories per Square Meter per Day		Calories per Square Foot per Day	
	Boys	Girls	Boys	Girls
1	1,140	1,110	106	103
2	1,150	1,090	107	101
3	1,130	1,040	105	96.6
4	1,100	1,020	102	94.8
5	1,070	998	99.4	92.7
6	1,050	989	97.5	91.9
7	1,030	970	95.7	90.1
8	1,010	960	93.8	89.2
9	998	948	92.7	88.1
10	979	890	90.9	82.7
11	937	960	87.0	89.2
12	1,150	960	107	89.2
13	1,100	936	102	87.0
14	1,080	936	100	87.0
15	1,080	840	100	78.0
16	1,070	792	99.4	73.6
17	1,050	775	97.5	72.0
18	1,030	773	95.7	71.8

* Adapted from Rose, Mary Swartz, *Foundations of Nutrition*, p. 101. By permission of The Macmillan Company, publishers.

Graph Showing Basal Energy Metabolism of Boys and Girls per Square Foot of Body Surface

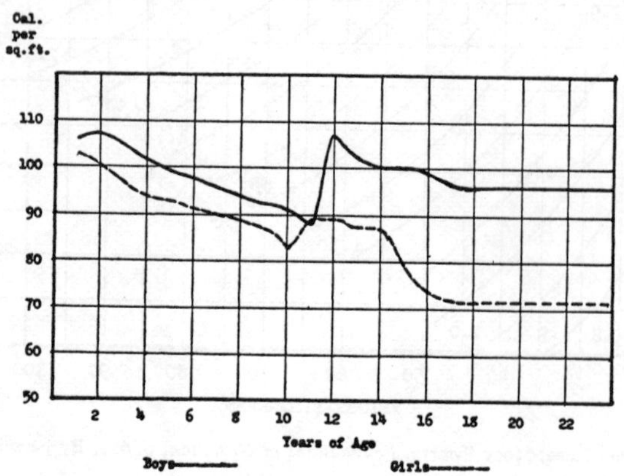

Basal Energy Metabolism of Children* in Terms of Body Weight

Age in Years	Calories per Pound per Day Boys	Girls
1	25	25
2	25	25
3	23	22
4	21	20
5	20	19
6	20	18
7	19	18
8	18	17
9	17	17
10	17	16
11	16	15
12	15	15
13	18	14
14	19	17
15	16	11
16	15	10
17	14	10

* Adapted from Rose, Mary Swartz, *Foundations of Nutrition*, p. 101. By permission of The Macmillan Company, publishers.

Graph Showing Basal Energy Metabolism of Children in Terms of Body Weight

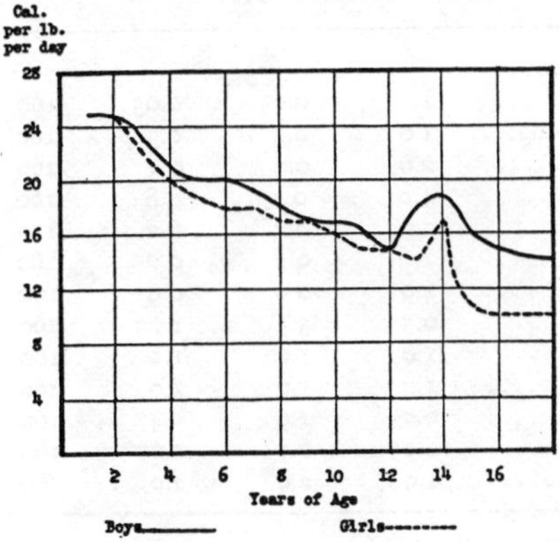

GRAPH SHOWING AVERAGE TOTAL DAILY ENERGY INTAKE OF NORMAL BOYS AND GIRLS (AFTER ROBERTS)*

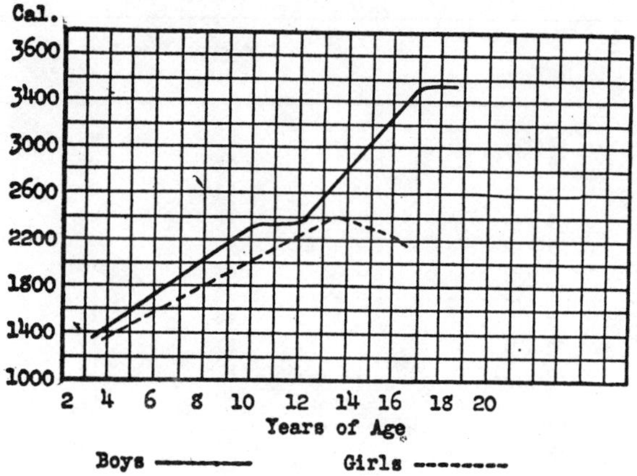

* From Rose, Mary Swartz, *Foundations of Nutrition*, p. 111. By permission of The Macmillan Company, publishers.

ANALYSIS OF ENERGY REQUIREMENT OF A 16-YEAR-OLD BOY WEIGHING 160 POUNDS

	Hours of Activity	Calories per Pound per Hour	Calories per Pound per Day	Pounds Body Weight	Total Expenditure per Day	Total Calories per Day
Basal requirement........	24.0		15.0	160	2,400.0	
Sleep..................	9.0	0.05	0.45	160	72.0	
Balance.................					2,328.0	2,328.0
Lying awake............	1.0	0.05	0.05	160	8.0	
Dressing and undressing...	1.0	0.3	0.3	160	48.0	
Eating.................	2.0	0.2	0.2	160	64.0	
Sitting.................	4.0	0.2	0.8	160	128.0	
Writing................	1.0	0.2	0.2	160	32.0	
Standing...............	1.0	0.2	0.2	160	32.0	
Walking................	1.0	0.9	0.9	160	144.0	
Running...............	0.5	3.3	1.65	160	264.0	
Bicycling..............	1.0	1.1	1.1	160	176.0	
Carpentry..............	1.0	1.0	1.0	160	160.0	
Walking downstairs.......	0.25	1.9	0.47	160	75.2	
Walking upstairs.........	0.25	6.7	1.67	160	267.2	
Playing ping-pong........	1.0	2.0	2.0	160	320.0	
Total cost of activities....					1,718.4	1,718.0
Total daily requirement...						4,046.0

GRAPH SHOWING ENERGY REQUIREMENT IN CALORIES OF A 16-YEAR-OLD BOY WEIGHING 160 POUNDS

(Each square represents 10 calories)

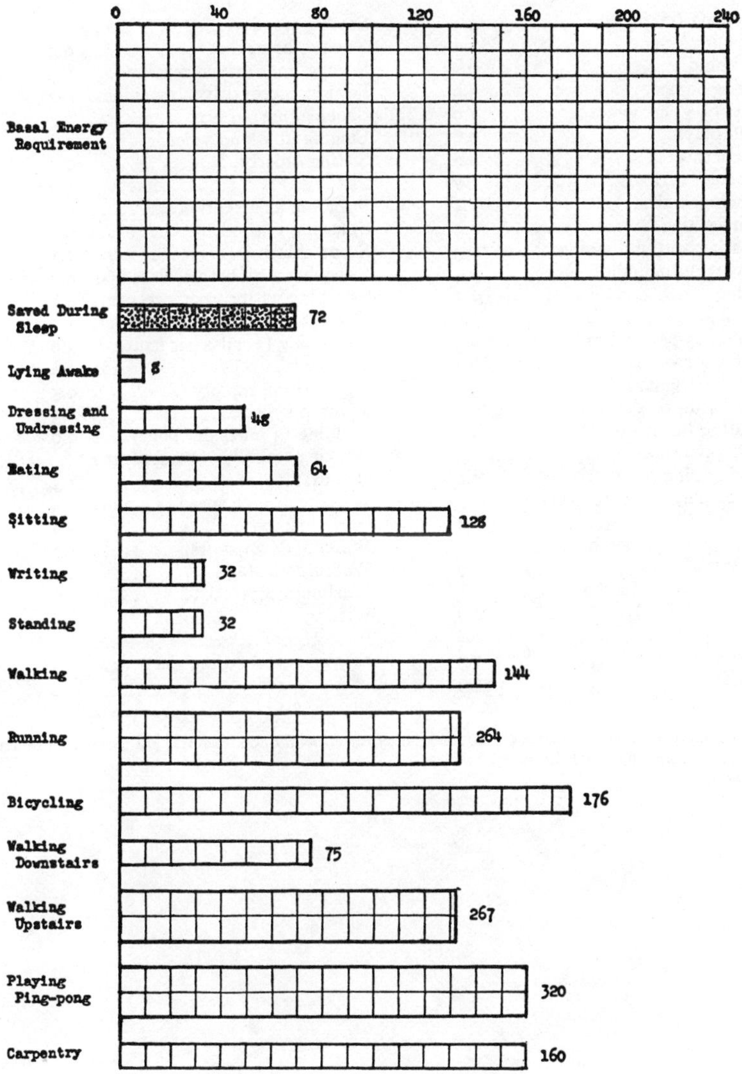

ENERGY COST OF ACTIVITIES*

Activity	Calories per Pound per Hour	Activity	Calories per Pound per Hour
Bicycling (racing)	3.4	Sawing wood	2.6
Bicycling (moderate speed)	1.1	Sewing, hand	0.2
Bookbinding	0.4	Sewing, foot driven machine	0.3
Boxing	5.0	Sewing, motor driven machine	0.2
Carpentry, heavy	1.0	Shoemaking	0.5
Cello playing	0.6	Singing in a loud voice	0.4
Crocheting	0.2	Sitting quietly	0.2
Dancing, foxtrot	1.7	Skating	1.6
Dancing, waltz	1.4	Standing at attention	0.3
Dishwashing	0.5	Standing relaxed	0.2
Dressing and undressing	0.3	Stone masonry	2.1
Driving automobile	0.4	Sweeping with broom, bare floor	0.7
Eating	0.2	Sweeping with carpet sweeper	0.8
Fencing	3.3	Sweeping with vacuum sweeper	1.2
Ironing (5-pound iron)	0.5	Swimming (2 miles per hour)	3.6
Knitting sweater	0.3	Tailoring	0.4
Laundry, light	0.6	Typewriting rapidly	0.5
Lying still, awake	0.5	Violin playing	0.3
Painting furniture	0.7	Walking (3 miles per hour)	0.9
Paring potatoes	0.3	Walking rapidly (4 miles per hour)	1.5
Playing ping pong	2.0	Walking at high speed (5.3 miles per hour)	3.8
Piano playing (Mendelssohn's "Songs")	0.4	Walking down stairs	1.9
Piano playing (Beethoven's "Appasionata")	0.7	Walking up stairs	6.7
Piano playing (Liszt's "Tarantella")	0.9	Washing floors	0.6
Reading aloud	0.2	Writing	0.2
Rowing in a race	7.3	Energy saved during sleep	0.05
Running	3.3		

* Adapted from Rose, Mary Swartz, *Foundations of Nutrition*, pp. 610-611. By permission of The Macmillan Company, publishers.

Dietary Standards in Shares for the Construction of Adequate Diets*

A *share* of any food nutrient represents 1/30 of the daily requirement of that nutrient for an adult using 3000 calories.
Thus:

One share of energy is 100 calories
One share of protein is 2.5 grams
One share of calcium is 0.023 gram
One share of phosphorus is 0.044 gram
One share of iron is 0.0005 gram
One share of vitamin A is 100 units (Sherman-Munsell)
One share of vitamin B is 10 units (Sherman-Chase)
One share of vitamin C is 2 units (Sherman-La Mer)
One share of vitamin G is 20 units (Sherman-Bourquin)

An adult should have one share of each dietary essential for each share of energy required. (Of course, the energy requirement is determined by the basal requirement and the activity of the individual).

DIETARY STANDARDS IN SHARES FOR HEALTHY ADULTS

Calories	Protein	Calcium	Phosphorus	Iron	Vitamin A	Vitamin B	Vitamin C	Vitamin G
24	24	24	24	24	24	24	24	24
25	25	25	25	25	25	25	25	25
26	26	26	26	26	26	26	26	26
27	27	27	27	27	27	27	27	27
28	28	28	28	28	28	28	28	28
29	29	29	29	29	29	29	29	29
30	30	30	30	30	30	30	30	30

High-school boys and girls have a similar standard with the exception that under no circumstances should they have less than 43 shares of calcium and 23 shares of phosphorus.

DIETARY STANDARDS IN SHARES FOR HIGH-SCHOOL BOYS AND GIRLS

Calories	Protein	Calcium	Phosphorus	Iron	Vitamin A	Vitamin B	Vitamin C	Vitamin G
20	20	43	23	20	20	20	20	20
23	23	43	23	23	23	23	23	23
25	25	43	25	25	25	25	25	25
30	30	43	30	30	30	30	30	30
35	35	43	35	35	35	35	35	35
40	40	43	40	40	40	40	40	40
43	43	43	43	43	43	43	43	43
45	45	45	45	45	45	45	45	45
50	50	50	50	50	50	50	50	50

* Adapted from Rose, Mary Swartz, *Foundations of Nutrition*, pp. 388; 600-601. By permission of The Macmillan Company, publishers.

GRAPH SHOWING DIETARY REQUIREMENTS IN SHARES FOR 16-YEAR-OLD BOY SPENDING 4046 CALORIES DAILY

(Each square represents 1 share)

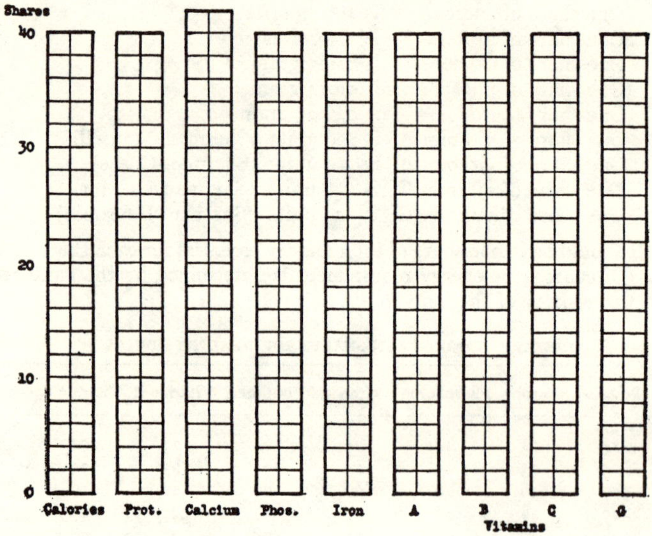

GRAPH SHOWING SHARES FURNISHED BY A 100 CALORIE PORTION OF MILK

(Each square represents 1 share)

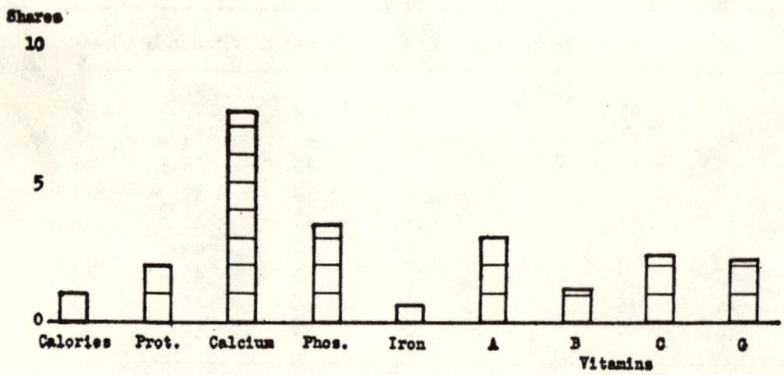

CONTRIBUTIONS OF FOOD TO THE DIET IN RELATION TO ENERGY VALUE*
(SHARE VALUES PER 100 CALORIES)

Food	Measure	Cal.	Pro.	Ca.	P.	Fe	A	B	C	G
CEREALS										
Bread, white	2 slices ½″ thick	1.0	1.4	0.5	0.8	0.7	—	?	—	—
Bread, whole wheat	2 slices	1.0	1.4	0.9	1.9	1.9	—	6.0	—	+
Oatmeal	¾ cup	1.0	1.7	0.7	2.3	1.9	+	6.0	—	+
Shredded wheat	1 bis.	1.0	1.4	0.5	2.0	2.5	—	6.0	—	+
Wheat germ	3 tbsp.	1.0	3.7	0.8	5.9	3.7	—	30.9	—	++
MILK										
Milk, whole	5/8 cup	1.0	1.9	7.6	3.1	0.7	3.2	1.6	2.5	2.2
FRUITS AND VEGETABLES										
Apples	1 large	1.0	0.3	0.5	0.5	1.0	0.9	+	6.5	1.9
Bananas	1 med.	1.0	0.5	0.4	0.7	1.2	3.6	2.9	8.5	1.8
Carrots	1 2/3 cups	1.0	1.0	5.4	2.3	2.7	101.4	6.4	7.0 R 4.5 CK	7.0
Lettuce	2 large heads	1.0	2.5	9.7	5.1	7.3	21.6	20.2	17.5	16.5
Oranges	1 large	1.0	0.6	3.8	0.9	0.8	1.8	7.7	57.5	4.1
Peas, green	¾ cup	1.0	2.8	1.1	2.9	3.3	6.6	22.0	26.5	5.0
Potatoes, white	1 med.	1.0	1.1	0.7	1.6	2.2	0.3	+	6.5	1.5
Raisins	2 tbsp.	1.0	0.3	0.8	0.9	1.2	1.1	2.4	—	—
Spinach	2½ cups 15 oz.	1.0	3.5	12.2	6.5	30.1	230.6	32.3	185.0 R 75.0 CN 14.0 CK	20.9
Tomatoes	3 med.	1.0	1.6	2.1	2.6	3.5	26.3	18.6	110.0 CN 110.0 CK	3.5
FATS										
Butter	1 tbsp.	1.0	0.1	—	—	—	4.3	—	—	—
Cottonseed oil	1 tbsp.	1.0	—	—	—	—	—	—	—	—
Oleomargarine	1 tbsp.	1.0	6.1	—	—	—	+	—	—	—
SUGARS										
Sugar	4 lumps	1.0	—	—	—	—	—	—	—	—
MEAT, FISH, EGGS, AND CHEESE										
Beef, lean	2.3 oz.	1.0	5.5	0.4	3.3	3.1	0.4	+	—	3.2
Eggs	1½ eggs	1.0	3.6	2.0	2.8	4.1	13.4	3.9	—	4.9
Liver	2.7 oz.	1.0	6.3	0.4	3.9	12.6	75.6	++	?	34.7

R—indicates raw. CN—indicates canned. CK—indicates cooked.

* Adapted from Rose, Mary Swartz, *Foundations of Nutrition*, pp. 560-599. By permission of The Macmillan Company, publishers.

Reference Books, Charts, and Bulletins

I. ESSENTIAL REFERENCE BOOKS

Peabody and Hunt. *Biology and Human Welfare.* (High school text) The Macmillan Company, 1933. $1.60.
Rose, Mary Swartz. *The Foundations of Nutrition.* (Revised Edition) The Macmillan Company, 1933. $3.00.
Rose, Mary Swartz. *Teaching Nutrition to Boys and Girls.* The Macmillan Company, 1932. $2.00.
Rose (M. S.) and Taylor (C. M.) *Food Values of Recipes in Shares and Vitamin Units.* Bureau of Publications, Teachers College, Columbia University, 1936. 35 cents.
Sherman, Henry C. *Food and Health.* The Macmillan Company, 1935. $2.50.

II. DESIRABLE REFERENCE BOOKS

Barber, Edith M. *What Shall I Eat?* The Macmillan Company, 1933. $2.00.
Bogert, L. Jean. *Diet and Personality.* The Macmillan Company, 1934. $2.00.
Bogert, L. Jean. *Nutrition and Physical Fitness.* W. B. Saunders Company, 1935. $3.00.
Charters, W. W., Smiley, Dean F., and Strang, Ruth M. *Health Through Science.* The Macmillan Company, 1935. $0.96. Also *The Body's Needs.* 1935. $0.92.
Diehl, Harold S. *Healthful Living.* McGraw-Hill Book Company, 1935. $2.50.
Dietz, David. *Medical Magic.* Dodd, Mead and Co., 1938. $3.50.
Fishbein, Morris, M. D. *Your Diet and Your Health.* McGraw-Hill Book Company, 1937. $2.50.
Furnas, C. C. and Furnas, S. M. *Man, Bread and Destiny.* Reynal and Hitchcock, 1937. $3.50.
Rose, Mary Swartz. *A Laboratory Handbook for Dietetics.* (Third Edition) The Macmillan Company, 1929. $3.00.
Adell, James C., Dunham, Orra Olive, and Welton, Louis E. *Explorations in Biological Science.* Ginn and Co., 1937.

III. USEFUL CHARTS AND BULLETINS

Building America, 425 West 123 Street, New York, N. Y.
"Food." 25 cents.
Burroughs Wellcome & Co., 9-11 East 41 Street, New York.
"Vitamins in Nutrition."
Carnegie Institution of Washington, Washington, D. C.
"Basal Metabolism."
"Birds as Heat Engines."
"Energy Consumption in Physical and Mental Effort."
"The Measure of Man's Vital Energy."
"Nutritional Improvement in Health and Longevity." (H. C. Sherman)
"Reptiles Used in Study of Human Physiology."
Dairy Council, Philadelphia, Pa.
Charts, pictures, and reference reading material assembled under the following topics: 1. Rocks and Soil; 2. The Growing Plant; 3. The Cow; 4. The Dairy Farm; 5. Transportation and Distribution; 6. Milk, the Food. $1.00.
Evaporated Milk Association, 203 North Wabash Avenue, Chicago.
"The Story of Evaporated Milk."

General Biological Supply House, Chicago.
"Laboratory Experiments in Nutrition." Turtox booklet. 1937. $1.00.
Metropolitan Life Insurance Co., 1 Madison Avenue, New York.
"The Family Food Supply."
"Three Meals a Day."
National Dairy Council, 111 North Canal Street, Chicago.
"Watch Them Grow." (Bulletin on rat experimentation)
United States Government Publications, Superintendent of Documents, Government Printing Office, Washington, D. C.
Charts 1-15. "Composition of Food Materials, etc." $1.50 per set.
Contents: 1. Milk and Milk Products; 2. Eggs and Cheese; 3. Meat, Fresh and Cured; 4. Fish, Fish Products, and Oysters; 5. Butter and Other Fat-yielding Foods; 6. Cereal Grains; 7. Bread and Other Cereal Foods; 8. Sugar and Similar Food; 9. Roots and Succulent Vegetables; 10: Legumes and Corn; 11. Fresh and Dried Fruits; 12. Fruit and Fruit Products; 13. Nuts and Nut Products; 14. Composition, Functions, and Uses of Food; 15. Dietary Standards.
Charts 1-8. "Food Selection and Meal Planning," showing week's supply of food for average family (2 adults and 3 children, or 4 adults). 50 cents per set.
"Diets of Low-Income Families Surveyed in 1933." (Public Health Reprint 1727) 5 cents.
"Diets to Fit the Family Income." 1936. (Farmers' Bulletin 1757) 5 cents.
"Effect of Cooking on Vitamin A and C Content of Fresh and Dried Apricots." 1933. (From *Journal of Agricultural Research*, Vol. 46, No. 9. Calif.-63). 5 cents.
"Eggs at Any Meal." (Agriculture Leaflet 39) 5 cents.
"Food for Children" (Farmers' Bulletin 1674) 5 cents.
"Good Food Habits for Children" (Agriculture Leaflet 42) 5 cents.
"Good Sources of Vitamins A and D." (Cooperative Extension Work) 5 cents.
"Good Sources of Vitamins B and C." (Cooperative Extension Work) 5 cents.
"Influence of Cooking and Canning on the Vitamin B and G Content of Lean Beef and Pork." (From *Journal of Agricultural Research*, Vol. 53, No. 6.) 5 cents.
"Milk for the Family." (Farmers' Bulletin 1705) 5 cents.
Nutrition charts 1-11. 50 cents per set.

1. "Growth as an Index of Nutrition." (White rats and other small animals are used for nutrition studies) 1934.
2. "Growth May Be Controlled by Diet." 1934.
3. "Protein for Building Muscle and Tissue." 1935.
4. "Calcium for Building Strong Bones and Teeth." 1934.
5. "Phosphorus Needed in All Parts of Body." 1934.
6. "Iron for Red Blood." 1934.
7. "Vitamin A for Growth, and Prevention of Certain Infections." 1934.
8. "Vitamin B for Good Appetite and Good Muscle Tone." 1934.
9. "Vitamin C for Healthy Gums and Teeth." 1935.
10. "Vitamin D for Good Bones and Teeth." 1935.
11. "Vitamin G for General Well-being." 1935.

"Vitamin A Content of Eggs Produced by Chickens Fed Viosterol and Various Percentages of Cod-liver Oil." 1935. (From *Journal of Agricultural Research*, Vol. 50, No. 10. T-7) 5 cents.

"Vitamin Content of Foods, Summary of Chemistry of Vitamins, Units of Measurement, Quantitative Aspects in Human Nutrition, and Occurrence in Foods." 1937. (Agriculture Misc. Publication 275) 20 cents.

University of Chicago Book Store, Chicago, Ill.

"Roberts Food Models." 75 cents.

University of Illinois, College of Agriculture, Urbana, Ill.

"Avitaminoses in Animals."

University of Wisconsin, Dept. of Dairy Industry, Madison, Wis.

"Light and Its Application to the Irradiation of Milk."

University of Wisconsin, Wisconsin Alumni Research Foundation, Bascom Hall, Madison, Wis.

Comparative Nutritional Chart.

Suggested Lesson Plans on the Vitamins A, B, C, D, E, G.

Testing Irradiated Evaporated Milk for Vitamin D.

Vitamin D Is Needed for Building Sound Teeth and Strong Bones.

What Happens When Foods Contain Too Little of Vitamins A, B, C, and G.

Why Irradiated Vitamin D Products Are Needed Most During Fall, Winter, Spring.

Construction and Use of Respiration Apparatus*

Little appreciation of the energy needs of the body can be achieved by high school pupils without some apparatus for measuring these energy needs. Standard equipment, such as that used in hospitals, is relatively expensive. A simple device, patterned after Benedict's Student Respiration Apparatus, can be constructed, which will enable pupils to make satisfactory determinations of their energy requirements when lying down or when sitting. It can also be used to show the energy cost of some activities.

Such an apparatus was recently constructed and used in the Demonstration High School of The Pennsylvania State College. The accompanying photograph shows some of the pupils of the biology class measuring the energy expenditure of one of their group. The diagram on page 58 shows the construction of the apparatus.

The materials used were:

A five-quart lubricating oil can
A small piece of inner tube rubber
A rubber shower hose
A bathing cap
Two glass Y tubes
Glass tubes for mouthpieces
Laboratory rubber tubing
A laboratory pump (bicycle pump is satisfactory)
Five pounds soda lime
Small tank of oxygen (desirable but not necessary)

The total cost of the apparatus was $3.89, and most of this cost went for the labor of the tinsmith who assembled the parts.

* This description of the construction and use of a respiration apparatus in one of the author's classes was first published in *The Science Leaflet*, Vol. X, No. 11, December 3, 1936.

The rubber valve was cut from an old inner tube, and held in place by the head of a shingle nail soldered to the valve seat. The top valve was constructed so that the rubber flap closed against the can, the lower so that the rubber flap closed against the end to which the rubber tube was attached. The curved wire was soldered on the side of the can to serve as a gauge for determining how high the rubber cap distended. The particular cap we used expanded sidewise, so we found it necessary to bend wires around the sides also. A metal shield was placed over the bottom valve to prevent soda lime from getting into it.

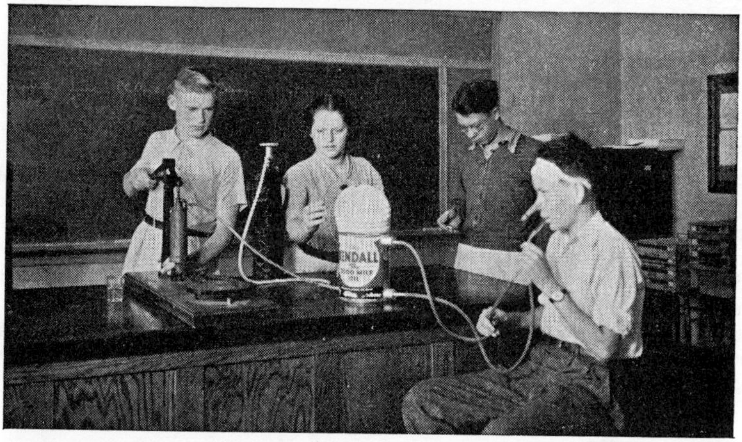

SHOWING THE USE OF THE RESPIRATION APPARATUS BUILT BY MEMBERS OF THE BIOLOGY CLASS, DEMONSTRATION HIGH SCHOOL, THE PENNSYLVANIA STATE COLLEGE, STATE COLLEGE, PENNSYLVANIA.

The first measurements were made with air alone. However, the subject felt he was not getting enough air for long, so the tests were limited to three minutes. Using oxygen made longer observations possible.

The pump for use in this experiment was calibrated by measuring the volume of air each pumpful would hold when such air was collected over a water bath by displacement of water from an inverted graduated cylinder.

To operate the homemade apparatus, one fills the container full of oxygen until the rubber cap touches the gauge wires at the sides and top. The subject then starts breathing. Time is counted from the first exhalation which fails to make the rubber cap touch the wires. The patient inhales air from the top of the container and exhales through the soda lime which absorbs carbon dioxide. Air is pumped in to replace the oxygen used by the subject. The operator adds just enough to make the cap touch the gauge wires each time the subject exhales as it did at the beginning. Record is kept of the number of pumpfulls consumed during the time of the test. The energy expenditure per day is calculated from these results by calculating the number of cubic centimeters of oxygen the subject would need per day and multiplying by the factor 0.004825. The tests gave the following results. Dean exercised vigorously during test number 10. The results seem quite plausible for high school boys and girls.

Case No.	Pump Fulls	Time in Min.	Cc. Oxygen Used	Cc. Oxygen per Day	Calories per Day
1. Jane...........	6	3	1290	619,200	2983
2. Stanley..........	8	3	1720	825,600	3984
3. Sylvia...........	5	3	1075	516,000	2490
4. Dean............	3	3	645	309,600	1493
5. Myra............	3	3	645	309,600	1493
6. Richard..........	6	3	1290	619,200	2983
7. Anna............	4	4	860	309,600	1493
8. Robert..........	6	5	1290	371,520	1796
9. Dean............	4	4	860	309,600	1493
10. Dean............	7	2½	1505	866,880	4183

This apparatus was later replaced by an improved model having larger air tubes and rubber "gas mask" valves. To assemble in this form, have a tinsmith make four smooth metal tubes 2½″ long and ¾″ in diameter, and one Y tube ¾″ in diameter. Solder two of the tubes on to the can as shown. With a cork borer drill holes in rubber stoppers so that one stopper can be placed on each metal tube. Put the rubber valves on the metal tubes so that air will pass from can to hose at top and from hose to can at bottom opening. Assemble glass housings over valves. Place 18″ length of hose on metal tube projecting from each valve. Attach rubber mouthpiece to the two rubber tubes by the metal Y tube.

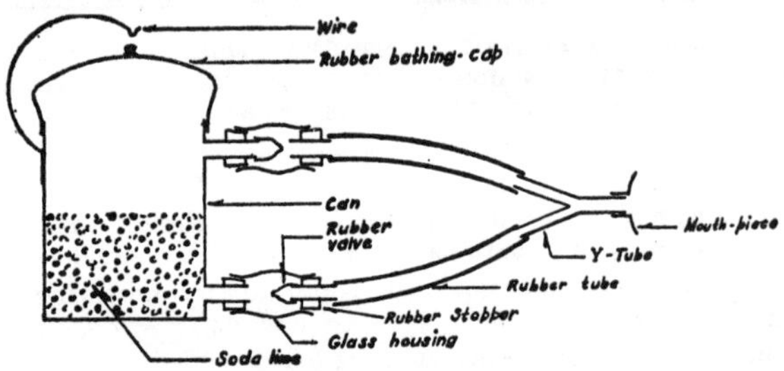

RESPIRATION APPARATUS

The cost of this assembly can be lessened by securing student lamp chimneys for use in place of glass housings.

Directions for Conducting Nutrition Experiments

Demonstration Diets*

For Rats

Control diet

	Gms.
Meat residue	20
Cornstarch	46
Butter	8
Cod liver oil	2
Salt mixture (O. & M.)†	4
Yeast (dried baker's)	20

Lacking vitamin B

	Gms.
Meat residue (B-free)	20
Cornstarch	46
Butter	8
Cod liver oil	2
Salt mixture (O. & M.)	4
Yeast (auto-claved baker's; i.e., heated at 110°C. for four hours)	20

Low calories

Feed these rats control diet (1) but limit their intake. About 0.12 gms. of food per gm. of rat per day should hold their weight nearly constant. (Or feed these animals 2/3 as much as control animals consume in terms of body weight.)

Stock diet for breeding rats

1/3 Klim (whole milk powder)
2/3 Whole wheat flour
2% Common salt

For Guinea Pigs

Lacking vitamin C

	Gms.
Mixture of rolled oats and bran (equal parts by volume)	59
Skim milk powder (heated 4 hrs. at 110°C)	30
Butter	10
Common salt	1

Adequate diet for guinea pig

Diet A with 10 gms. of spinach, potato, or 1.0 mg. of pure vitamin C daily.

Making Meat Residue Vitamin Free for Experiments

(12 pounds of meat will fill a 2-quart can with residue)

1. Procure 3 lbs. very lean—finest chopped—round steak.
2. Heat water in 4-qt. pan to boiling.
3. Drop meat in hot water.
4. Heat to boiling and boil for 5 minutes.
5. Pour off all possible fat from top.
6. Strain rest through double thickness cheesecloth—squeeze.
7. Regrind meat in meat grinder.
8. Repeat 2 to 7 twice more.
9. Dry in shallow trays in electric oven at 60° C.
10. Pulverize with coffee grinder.

* Diets used by Professors Rose and McCloud in Nutrition Laboratory, Teachers College, Columbia University, N. Y. C.

† The Osborne and Mendel salt mixture contains all the mineral elements required by the rat; viz., calcium, magnesium, sodium, potassium, phosphorus, chlorine, sulphur, iron, iodine, and manganese.

Care of Animals

1. Daily care:
   a. Change papers under cages.
   b. Salvage unspoiled food and return to food cup.
   c. If food is needed, weigh out enough (50 to 100 grams) to last several days and record amount given on a card. (This record is optional but interesting if time permits.)
   d. Use every precaution not to mix rats or diets. One wrong feeding can upset results.
   e. Fill water cups with fresh clean water.
   f. Record any noticeable changes in appearance of animals.
2. Weighing day (Rats should be weighed each week at same time):
   a. Weigh each rat and record weight on card and on graph.
   b. (If keeping record of food consumed.) Weigh food left in cup. From this, calculate food consumed per cage per day and per gram of rat per day.
3. Graphic weight records (Make on ¼ inch cross section paper):
   a. Make crosswise of paper. (The suggestion is made that you plot the rat weights against the normal rate of growth given on page 61). Use one sheet of graph paper for each cage.
   b. Scale for weight curve:
      (1) For rats:
         2 sq. horizontally—1 week.
         1 sq. vertically—10 grams body weight.
      (2) For guinea pigs start scale at 160 grams.
   c. Indicate changes in diet by an arrow and footnote.
4. Miscellaneous notes:
   a. Rats should all be the same age. From three to four weeks is best age.
   b. Guinea pigs should weigh about 250 grams at beginning of experiment. Feed both cages on adequate diet until they weigh about 300 grams; then start one cage on deficient diet.
   c. One kilogram of food is enough for two rats for six weeks.
   d. Animals should not be subject to drafts or extreme changes in temperature.
   e. Rose* gives much interesting information about experimentation with rats for school purposes.
   f. Approximate food requirements of control rats per week:

Weeks of Age	Food per Cage in Grams	Grams of Food per Gram of Rat
4	67.	0.84
5	97.	0.84
6	126.	0.84
7	145.	0.77
8	160.	0.70
9	170.	0.63
10	168.	0.56

* Rose, Mary Swartz, *Teaching Nutrition to Boys and Girls*, Appendix. By permission of the Macmillan Company, publishers.

Normal Growth Curve of Rats on Stock Diet "F" Above

An excellent way of plotting the growth of each cage of experimental animals which you keep is as follows. Take ¼″ cross section paper 8½ x 11 for each cage of rats, in which you would likely have a male and a female experimental animal. Plot the normal growth curve for both the male and female in dotted lines, using the scale indicated on page 60. Then plot the weight of your experimental animals, male and female, in solid lines. By such a procedure it is possible to compare your control animals and your experimental animals against the normal growth curve. This curve has been established through records kept on hundreds of animals. The following are the data of a normal curve for growth of rats on stock diet given on page 59.*

Age in Weeks	Male Weight in Grams	Female Weight in Grams	Age in Weeks	Male Weight in Grams	Female Weight in Grams
4............	40	40	15..........	230	172
5............	58	58	16..........	238	178
6............	78	72	17..........	245	185
7............	100	88	18..........	252	190
8............	124	104	19..........	258	192
9............	147	122	20..........	265	196
10............	164	136	21..........	271	199
11............	182	150	22..........	278	202
12............	199	158	23..........	282	204
13............	212	162	24..........	285	205
14............	223	167	on..........	285	205

Normal Growth Curve for Rats

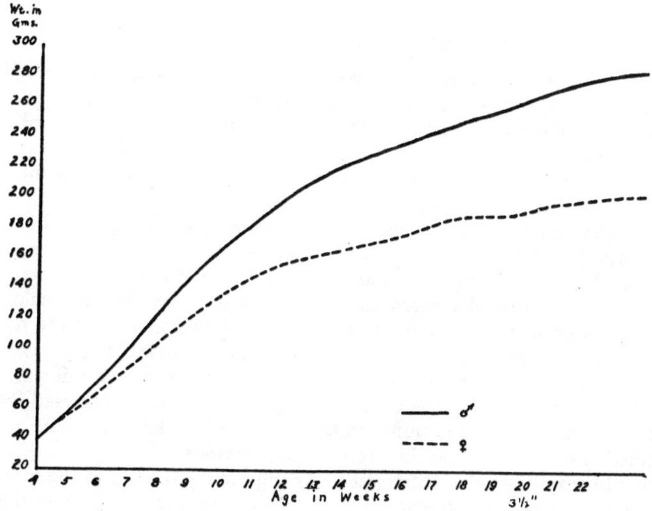

* Adapted from Rose, Mary Swartz, *Teaching Nutrition to Boys and Girls*, Appendix. By permission of The Macmillan Company, publishers.

Construction of Cages

Suitable cages can be made from ⅜″ or ½″ mesh hardware cloth and two shallow pans or flat pieces of board or metal which serve as bottom and top. This hardware cloth costs approximately 7 cents per square foot, making the cost for each about 30 cents. Cut the strips of hardware cloth as indicated in the two diagrams. After cutting, bend the projections on the disc in one direction so that they will serve as legs to support the floor of the cage. Wrap the rectangular piece of hardware cloth around this floor, lace the ends of the rectangular piece together with fine wire, and lace the floor in place with fine wire. This cage can then be set on a newspaper in a shallow pan or on flat pieces of board. Tops can be made of shallow pans or small boards any of which can be weighted down with a brick or stone. Laboratory beakers can easily be wired in place for water dishes and feeding dishes. (The ends of orange boxes make excellent tops and bottoms for cages.)

Way to Cut Hardware Cloth When Making Cages

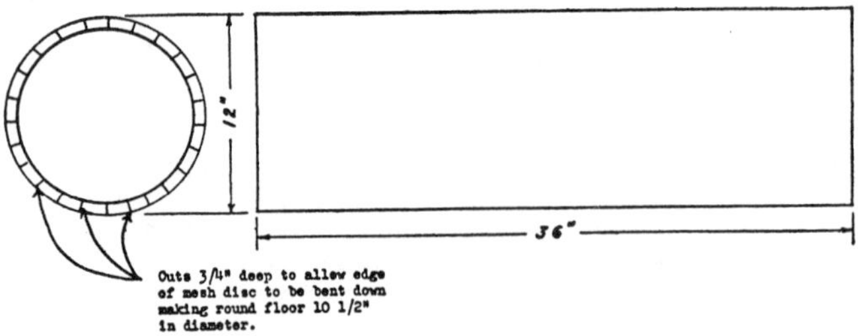

White Rats as Laboratory Animals*

The following is quoted from "Animal Experiments Conducted at the Nutrition Laboratory Battle Creek Sanitarium," by Dr. Helen S. Mitchell.

One of the first questions asked by a new visitor in the laboratory is "Why do you use rats for this work?" The answer is simply that there is no other animal which can so well meet the needs of the laboratory worker in this field. A rat will eat almost any human food, his digestive tract is similar to man's, he is comparatively free from infectious disease if properly cared for, and his short life cycle makes possible observations over several generations if this is desirable. Rats from the same litter grow at approximately the same rate and so serve admirably for comparison of contrasting diets. All animals in the same colony under the same environment show similar rates of growth and it is therefore possible to establish a normal growth curve for the males and females in any given colony which may be used for comparison with growth curves of other animals from the same colony stunted by various food deficiencies. The young rats used for experimental work are all raised in our own laboratory where known conditions can be maintained through the gestation and nursing periods.

The life history of a rat is interesting as compared with that of the human, and certain comparisons may be made more rationally by the use of these figures:

* From *Popular Survey*, 1927. (Out of print.)

Weight of rat at birth	1/6 to 1/5 oz.
Number of young in a litter	4 to 13; av. 7 or 8
Gestation period	3 weeks
Nursing period	3 to 4 weeks
Weight at weaning	1 to 1 2/3 oz.
Rapid growing period	Birth to 5 months
Sex mature	3 months
Length of life	2 to 3 years
Weight at 5 months	Males 10½ oz. Females 6½ oz.

One year in a rat's life may in some respects be considered equivalent to 30 years in a human, and certain food requirements also seem to stand in about the ratio of 1 to 30.

Sources of Supplies with Approximate Costs

I. SOURCES

1. Breeding and Laboratory Institute, 619 Kent Ave., Brooklyn, N. Y. Animals, cages, etc.
2. Collins, Warren E., 555 Huntington Ave., Boston, Mass. Respiration apparatus accessories.
3. Eimer and Amend, 18th St. and 3rd Ave., New York, N. Y. Chemicals, rubber tubing, stoppers, and other apparatus.
4. General Biological Supply House, 761-763 East 69th Place, Chicago, Ill. Animals, diets, cages, nutrition booklet, apparatus, etc.
5. Ralston Purina Company, St. Louis, Mo. Complete rations for laboratory animals; booklet on care of animals.
6. The Albino Supply Company, Philadelphia, Pa. White rats.
7. The Harris Laboratories, Inc., Tuckahoe, N. Y. Experimental diets, materials for diets, diets to order.

II. APPROXIMATE COSTS

1. Feeding experiments:

a. 3-4-week old rats	35¢-50¢ each
b. 250-gram guinea pigs	50¢-75¢ each
c. 275-gram pigeons	50¢-75¢ each
d. Sufficient diet for cage of experimental animals	$1.25-$1.75
e. Material for cages	30¢ each
f. Approximate total cost for each cage of two animals	$2.00-$2.25

Suggest the following five cages of experimental animals:

(1) Cage of two rats on control diet.
(2) Cage of two rats on low calorie diet.
(3) Cage of two rats on vitamin B deficient diet.
(4) Cage of one or two guinea pigs on control diet.
(5) Cage of one or two guinea pigs on vitamin C deficient diet.

2. Home-made respiration apparatus.......................... $4.00-$15.00

   a. From Warren E. Collins:
      1 nose clip.. $1.25
      1 mouthpiece.. 1.00
      2 glass housings for valves.. 4.50
      2 rubber valves for respiration apparatus.. 1.00
      1 bathing cap with button attached.. 1.25
      1 rubber band to hold bathing cap.. .25

   b. From Eimer and Amend:
      3 feet 30692 best black heavy wall rubber tubing, inside diameter ¾".. $1.80
      4 No. 7, 1 hole rubber stoppers.. .40
      5 pounds soda lime, 4-8 mesh.. 2.25

3. Reference books, charts, and bulletins.......................... $10.00-$15.00

CHAPTER IV

Tests Used in the Experiment

THREE tests were constructed for use in the experiment. The first was constructed to measure the pupils' attitude toward the selection of food. This test was made in two forms. The form used at the Lincoln School in the first experiment was entitled "How I Select My Diet." The form used in the extended experiment was entitled "The Way I Live." The change in form was made to camouflage the purpose of the test. The second test was constructed to measure the pupils' understanding of nutrition. It was of the true-false type and was entitled "Information Test." The third test was designed to measure the pupils' application of knowledge in the interpretation of statements in current advertisements. This test was entitled "Advertisement Interpretation Test." The same form of each test was used as an initial test and again as a final test.

The reasons for selecting the above areas for measurement and the steps followed in the construction of the instruments are given below. Copies of the tests, together with scoring keys, are included. The attitudes test is treated first, the information test second, and the application test last.

Since no suitable tests were available the problem became one of determining the characteristics one wished to study and then of constructing tests to measure them. Symonds[1] states that "the first concern of one who wishes to choose a standardized test is to make sure that it really measures what it purports to measure. The adequacy and detail with which a test is a measure of a treated function or school subject is called its validity." This criterion should apply equally well to the choice of standardized tests or to the construction of tests.

What characteristics should be studied? If this nutrition work belongs in high school classes, it not only should give pupils increased

[1] Symonds, *Measurement in Secondary Education,* p. 279.

knowledge concerning the foods they eat, but should also function in their daily lives. To be of value in improving their health it should affect their daily selection of food. It seemed to the investigator that he might measure the pupils' intelligent concern about foods by constructing an attitudes test somewhat after the pattern used by Thurstone and Chave.[2] Thus he set out to construct a test to measure pupils' attitudes concerning the relation of food to their well-being, as expressed in the choice of their daily menu. This test in its first form was called "How I Select My Diet"; in the final form it was called "The Way I Live."

Of course it was necessary to know whether or not pupils having this experience gained in their knowledge and understanding of the field of nutrition. This required some type of subject-matter test, and a true-false test, called "Information Test," was selected as most appropriate for the purpose.

In addition, the investigator wished to devise some measure of pupils' ability to apply principles and understandings to everyday situations. One test was constructed in an attempt to measure their use of knowledge in interpreting situations in their environment. This test, which was called an "Advertisement Interpretation Test," asked pupils to pass judgment on the truth or falsity of statements excerpted from food advertisements in current magazines.

CONSTRUCTING THE ATTITUDES TEST

In constructing the attitudes test, "The Way I Live," the following questionnaire was devised to stimulate biology pupils to write statements concerning the way they select their diet.

Personal Reactions to Nutrition Problems

I need to collect a list of statements about the way people feel concerning the diets they eat and how they select these diets. I should appreciate your describing in short statements your feelings or actions in regard to the following.

1. How do you judge the eating places where you dine?
2. How do you select your meals when eating out?
3. How does attractiveness enter into what you eat?
4. How do "vitamins" enter into the selection of what you eat?
5. How do you determine how much you will eat?
6. How does "fattening" enter into your choice of foods?

[2] Thurstone, L. L. and Chave, E. J., *Measurement of Attitude.*

7. How does "laxative" enter into your choice of foods?
8. How does "rich in calcium" enter into your choice of foods?
9. How does "delicious" enter into your choice of foods?
10. How does "most for your money" enter into your choice of foods?
11. How does "is good for me" enter into your choice of foods?
12. To what extent do you select uncooked vegetable or leafy salads? Why?
13. To what extent do you select tomato juice or orange juice? Why?
14. To what extent do you select milk in your diet? Why?
15. To what extent do you select whole-wheat cereals and breadstuffs? Why?
16. What should one be most concerned about in selecting a place to dine in addition to cleanliness?
17. Does one's diet have much to do with daily efficiency?
18. What relation, if any, exists between one's diet and his tendency to catch cold?
19. What, if any, relation exists between one's diet and his ability to recover speedily from illness?
20. How do you feel about paying attention to the calories in foods?
21. How do you feel about paying attention to the vitamins in foods?
22. Is dieting foolishness or good sense? Why?
23. Is it dangerous to diet? Why or why not?
24. If one diets, how should he do it?
25. Is fatness largely the result of carelessness about what one eats or does it just run in families?
26. How important is it for one to have a quart of milk a day?
27. Suppose that one eats what he wants, will his appetite take care of him?
28. Should the diet of an athlete or that of a writer be the more carefully selected? Why?
29. What are the most important things to consider in selecting one's diet?
30. Should one have pastry or cake each day? Why or why not?

This questionnaire was given to about fifty biology pupils in one of the New York City public schools, and from the statements they gave over six hundred statements were collected. The investigator wished to get statements phrased in the language used by high school boys and girls in order to increase the validity of the scale. From these statements were selected 135 which seemed to state rather clearly a definite position in reference to the selection of one's diet. Next, a group of adults were asked to go over the items and to check them for clarity, simplicity, and meaningfulness.

How could these items be rated so that agreement with them in a test would indicate concern or lack of concern about the healthful qualities of food? Using a simplification of the technique described by Thurstone and Chave, twenty-five persons, some experts in nutrition, some graduate students, others lay people, were asked to sort these items according to the directions below:

Attached are several statements, most of which have been made by high school boys and girls, which reflect their attitude with regard to the selection of foods.

I should like to use many of these statements in the construction of an attitude scale. The attitude scale ranges from complete disregard for the healthful qualities when selecting one's foods, to careful selection of one's foods on the basis of their contribution to one's health.

Please help to construct the scale as follows:

1. Sort the statements into three groups: group A, indicating more disregard than regard for healthful qualities of foods; group B, indicating about equal concern and unconcern for the healthful qualities of foods; group C, indicating more concern about the healthful qualities than other matters when selecting foods.
2. Sort group A into two groups: group 1, those which express absolutely no concern about the healthful qualities of foods; group 2, those which indicate a slight concern about the healthful qualities of foods.
3. Sort group C into two groups: group 1, those which have considerable concern about the healthful qualities of foods; group 2, those which indicate selection of their foods primarily on the basis of the healthful qualities in them.

A frequency distribution was made of the opinions of these judges as to whether or not each item expressed much, moderate, neutral, slight, or a lack of concern about the healthful qualities of foods selected. From this frequency distribution it was possible to select twenty items for each of the five statements on which there was marked agreement by the judges. This made a total of one hundred items, which were assembled in a test and tried out experimentally with two high school classes in a neighboring school. These classes were asked to check the statements with which they agreed and to disregard the others.

These results were scored according to an arbitrary scale from 1 to 5, giving one point for each item checked at the low end of the scale and five points for each item checked at the high end of the scale. Total scores were secured for each pupil taking the test. These total scores were arranged in rank order. Items which did not distinguish between those pupils having the best attitude as expressed in terms of their selection of diet and the poorest attitude as expressed in terms of their selection of diet were obviously of little value for the scale. Hence, the total number of responses made by the upper quartile and the lower quartile of the class on each item was determined. Those items which did not distinguish between the upper quartile and the lower quartile were discarded. This left eighty items which seemed to have some value for the scale.

In order further to validate the position of these eighty items, the scale was again referred to twenty-five seniors at the Lincoln School, who were asked to judge the items exactly as had been done before. Thus was provided a total of fifty judgments on each item. Each stage had twenty items. In order to determine the reliability of the test, ten items in each stage were matched as nearly as possible against the ten other items, producing two approximately equal halves. These eighty items were then shuffled and arranged in a scale for use in the first experiment. Pupils were asked to check the scale according to these directions: "Following are several statements reflecting how different people select the foods they eat. You will find that you agree with some and disagree with others. Place a check after those with which you agree. Probably you will not agree with more than fifteen or twenty of the statements included."

The test in this form revealed a considerable difference between the experimental group and the control group at the Lincoln School. However, some members of the class seemed to check a large percentage of the items, while other members checked very few. Possibly the few who tended to check a large percentage of the items could be made more discriminating by giving them an opportunity to check each item. Hence the form was revised by asking pupils to check each statement in an "agree" column, a "question" column, or a "disagree" column. This technique tended to limit the range of agreement.

What certainty was there that the pupils were not agreeing with the statements with which they believed their teacher wanted them to agree? In other words, was the test measuring their attitude toward the selection of diet, or was it measuring their ability in selecting teacher-approved answers? This challenge could not go unheeded, and so the test was revised to its present form, camouflaging teacher-purpose by inserting a larger number of extraneous items than test items. This meant a careful selection of the more discriminating scale items, and the formulating of items for camouflage in the same style as those used as test items. Such camouflaged items were arranged to express lack of concern or deep concern toward exercise, toward selection of clothing, toward personal hygiene, toward posture, toward recreation, toward rest, and toward social relations. These extraneous items were then shuffled with forty items selected from the original test. The test was used in this form for an extended experiment in 1937.

In order to make certain that the test was measuring the pupil's attitude as expressed in his daily selection of diet, permission was granted to give the test to a group of twenty graduate students in an advanced nutrition course. Certainly the concern in the selection of diet by these mature students who are making nutrition a life profession should be of the highest type. According to this criterion the test was valid, as is shown by the fact that this group far outranked the experimental group even after the latter had had instruction.

There were, however, a few items upon which the nutrition experts did not agree. It was suggested that a more valid rating scale be devised in terms of the agreement of the twenty experts checking the items. These judges showed considerable agreement when checking thirty-one out of the forty items. This agreement, together with the points of credit assigned each item, is shown in the succeeding array:

Number of Judges Agreeing on a Given Item	Number of Items on Which Judges Agreed			Points of Credit Assigned Each Item	Cumulative Points of Credit Assigned		
	Agree Items	Disagree Items	All Items		Agree Items	Disagree Items	All Items
20	7	2	9	4	28	8	36
19	6	3	9	4	24	12	36
18	1	2	3	3	3	6	9
17	2	1	3	2	4	2	6
16	3	0	3	2	6	0	6
15	0	3	3	2	0	6	6
14	1	0	1	1	1	0	1
Totals	20	11	31		66	34	100

Thus if nineteen or twenty of these experts checked an "agree" or "disagree" item, four points of credit were assigned to that item; if eighteen of the experts checked an "agree" or "disagree" item, three points were given for that item; if fifteen to seventeen, two points; and if fourteen, one point. Thus was provided a scale of one hundred points on which to rate the test, with eighteen four-point statements, three three-point statements, nine two-point statements, and one one-point statement. Lorge[3] found this technique of giving credit to both "agree" and "disagree" items to be satisfactory. There is a high correlation between a pupil's tendency to disagree with a discriminating item and his total score on a test, as well as a high correlation between his tendency to agree with a discriminating item and his total score.

The correlations computed on the scores made by the thirty-two pupils of the first experimental group at the Lincoln school were:

.901 between "agree" score and "total" score
.996 between "disagree" score and "total" score
.774 between "agree" score and "disagree" score

All three correlations are significantly different from zero.[4] Scores made on the "agree" items measure the same characteristics that are measured by the "total" score.

The first experimental group marked "agree" items only.[5] Their papers were re-scored on the "agree" items in accordance with the judgment of the experts.[6] The total score possible on the "agree" items was sixty-six points.

The test items in the revised form were then paired to determine the reliability.[7] The two halves compared thus:

	One Half	Other Half
Number of items................	16	15
Number of "agree" items.........	10	10
Number of "disagree" items.......	6	5
Number of points of credit........	50	50

The final form of the test, "The Way I Live," as given during the extended experiment follows immediately (page 72).

[3] Irving Lorge, Teachers College, Columbia University; unpublished research.

[4] Fisher's 5 per cent level of significance is .349; his 1 per cent level is .449. Fisher, R. A., *Statistical Methods for Research Workers.* 1937.

[5] Cf. page 9.

[6] Cf. page 70.

[7] Cf. page 84.

Test No. 1. Attitudes Test: "The Way I Live"

Directions. Following are several statements reflecting how different people live. You will find that you agree with some of the statements and disagree with others. Place a check in the column headed (A) if you agree with the statement or practice. Place a check in the column headed (D) if you disagree with the statement or practice. If you neither agree nor disagree with the statement or practice or are indifferent to it place a check in the column headed (?). *Be sure to mark each item.* The following example illustrates the method of marking:

Example:

	A	?	D
1. I try to get to school on time.	√		
2. I prefer shabby clothes to smart clothes.			√
3. I prefer hard work to play. .		√	

	A	?	D
1. I seldom, if ever, participate in strenuous outdoor exercise.			
2. A poor posture may keep one from doing his best in his studies.			
3. I do not select clothes for style only.			
4. I do the things I wish to do regardless of what the other boys and girls my age are doing.			
5. I am never concerned whether or not a food is good for me			4*
6. I try to build up a good body reserve of strength by having a good diet.	4		
7. I believe the food I eat has very little to do with the condition of my skin.			
8. I select any food which looks good to me.			2
9. I believe I can judge what is best for me no matter what others may be doing.			
10. I never think of the calories in foods.			3
11. Sometimes I prefer to be with a group of my friends; at other times I prefer to be alone.			
12. I try to select a nourishing meal for as little cost as possible	2		
13. In my opinion the balanced diets commonly advertised have the vitamins in sufficiency so I may forget about them.			4
14. I prefer clothes like those worn by my best friends.			
15. I think daily outdoor exercise would be good for me. . . .			
16. If I were overweight I am sure I should diet.	2		
17. I prefer to do exciting things so play few games.			
18. Clothes are individual, and should, I believe, be chosen to suit one's personality.			
19. I try to get outdoor exercise every day.			

* The numbers in the columns show points of credit assigned.

	A	?	D
20. I drink milk because I think it is good for me.	4		
21. I select my foods to avoid sluggishness.	2		
22. Occasionally I get outdoor exercise by walking or skating			
23. I prefer movies and similar types of entertainment to games and sports.			
24. I see to it that I get regular and sufficient rest with no two late nights in succession.			
25. I make it a point to get outdoor exercise daily except in inclement weather.			
26. I select my food so that I shall have a variety of vitamins in my diet.	4		
27. I select milk frequently because it is one of our most nutritive foods.	4		
28. My chief consideration in choosing clothes is style.			
29. I usually take a shower after strenuous exercise.			
30. I see to it that I get some form of recreation daily, preferably out-of-doors.			
31. I consider the effect of foods on health when selecting my meals.	4		
32. I do not care what I eat as long as it is good.			2
33. It is best not to embarrass others at a party by refraining from drinking and smoking.			
34. I have regular hours for going to bed.			
35. I select some foods to maintain my efficiency.	4		
36. I do not consider the effect of foods on my body when selecting them.			4
37. I so plan my recreation that it yields both present pleasure and future benefit.			
38. I think one is a poor sport to refrain from drinking and smoking when others are doing it.			
39. I drink a glass per day of orange or tomato juice to keep up on vitamins.	2		
40. Some people should consider calories in selecting their food.	4		
41. I select milk, cheese, and dairy products for their food value to me.	4		
42. I see to it that I get plenty of minerals.	4		
43. I have several hobbies which are very challenging to me			
44. I usually stay with my group of friends even though I am not interested in what they are doing.			
45. I do not bathe any oftener than I have to in order to look clean.			
46. I maintain an excellent body carriage for it improves both my appearance and my efficiency.			
47. I see no relationship between my posture and my general well-being.			

	A	?	D
48. I do not need to worry about my food if I select the things I want from the menus commonly served			2
49. I select wholesome and tasty meals	4		
50. If one leads an active life he need not worry about his posture			
51. I prefer vitamin rich foods, but am not fanatical on the subject	3		
52. I am sure it is essential to my well-being to have a variety of foods in my diet	4		
53. I try to take a good posture when I think of it, but old habits usually get the best of me			
54. I select my meals on the basis of wholesomeness and healthful qualities	4		
55. If clothes are expensive and not durable, I will not choose them even though my best friends may			
56. I am frequently up late at night			
57. A little drinking and smoking will not hurt me if others are doing it			
58. I determine my eating places on the basis of good reputation	1		
59. If I were fat I should try to reduce by eating less rich food	4		
60. I seldom choose to eat raw vegetables			3
61. I seldom take more than one dessert even though I should enjoy having it	2		
62. Frequently I am up late two or three nights in succession			
63. My daily work requires skill and concentration so I plan to refrain from drinking and smoking			
64. It should be a requirement for graduation that all of us take proper care of our bodies and correct all the defects we can			
65. I never give vitamins a thought			4
66. I believe a healthy body promotes a healthy skin			
67. I think it is sensible to plan on getting plenty of rest			
68. I plan to participate in some strenuous physical activities each week			
69. Food seems to have very little effect upon my daily efficiency			4
70. Thinking about the calories in foods is not practical for everyday eating			2
71. I always like to do what my friends are doing			

CONSTRUCTING THE INFORMATION TEST

To construct the information test, called "Test No. 2, Information Test," every effort was made to have the test items parallel closely the emphasis given to the subject as studied in the experimental situation. Symonds states that "in the case of achievement tests most of the validation of the tests can be accomplished by the original choice of material for the test." [8]

The sampling seemed to group itself into twenty-three definite groups. From four to seven questions were set up for each of these groups. Care was used to see that there were an equal number of true and false items, and the material was checked to remove as many ambiguous and meaningless statements as possible. However, several indiscriminate questions remained, some long, some trivial, some suggestive, and some with dependent clauses, some containing separate ideas either of which may be false, and a few containing specific determiners such as "always," "never," and "only."

Since the time available to the examiner allowed for the administration of seventy-five to one hundred items, the test was begun with one hundred seventy-five items in the trial form, with the thought that much improvement could be gained by discarding the non-discriminatory items. The test was then given to a group of about thirty biology pupils in a neighboring school. The scores made by these pupils were ranked and the upper quartile and the lower quartile were determined. Then the responses made by the upper quartile and the lower quartile on each item were plotted. Most of those items which failed to distinguish between the lower quartile and upper quartile were discarded as inferior. However, a few items which belonged with the subject matter not previously covered by any of the trial group were included even though they were entirely omitted by the majority of both the upper and the lower quartiles. Also, several adults checked through the test and searched for items which should be discarded. As a result of these crude methods of refinement, a test of ninety true-false items closely paralleling the understandings to be taught was constructed. This test was used in the first experiment. At the end of the first experiment it appeared that some of the emphases made in the treatment should be modified before extending the experiment to include other schools. This meant that it was necessary to drop a few test items and substitute others paralleling them.

As a further guarantee of its validity the refined test was also given to the group of twenty advanced nutrition students who examined the attitudes test. The results were checked against the scoring

[8] Symonds, Percival, *Measurement in Secondary Education,* p. 280.

key and those items with which the majority of the judges did not agree were discarded in the final scoring. This left seventy-eight items in the test used for the extended experiment in 1937. Sixty-three of these items were identical with those used in the first experiment and it seemed wise, in interpreting the first experiment, to base the results upon these valid items. Twenty of the experts agreed with fifteen of the seventy-eight items; nineteen with twelve; eighteen with fifteen; seventeen with thirteen; sixteen with six; fifteen with five; fourteen with five; thirteen with five; and twelve with two. This means that the knowledge and understandings, as scored in "Information Test," are in accordance with the opinion of experts, and hence valid.

The test items were then divided into halves by the odd and even method for the determination of reliability.[9]

Test No. 2. Information Test

Directions. Following are several statements. Some are true, others are false. If any part of a statement is wrong it should be considered false. If a statement is true, place a plus sign (+) in the corresponding blank space to the right of the statement. If a statement is false place a minus sign (−) in the corresponding blank space to the right of the statement. Do not guess. The following example illustrates the way to mark the test:

Example: It snows more frequently
  a. in winter than in summer.......... 1. +
  b. in summer than in winter.......... 2. −

1. The study of nutrition should be of value because:
   a. the majority of us are taking in more calories than we need 1. −*
   b. the majority of us are enjoying normal health which could be changed to buoyant health by attention to our diet......... 2. +
   c. an individual can select the diets best for himself by being thoroughly informed about the problem of nutrition......... 3. +
   d. sales pressure through advertising tends to modify our food selection.. 4. +

2. We can effectively study diets in the following ways:
   a. have part of our class eat one diet and have another part eat another diet.. 5. −
   b. secure suitable laboratory animals, feed one pair a known good diet and the other pair a similar diet with a known food essential eliminated.. 6. +

[9] Cf. page 84. * + and − indicate correct answers.

c. feed two young female rats a good diet and two young male rats a similar diet with a known food essential eliminated.... 7. –

3. The total amount of energy which the body expends is greater for:
   a. a growing boy of kindergarten age than for a high-school boy 8. –
   b. a 140-pound man when doing work than for a 140-pound high-school boy doing the same work........................ 9. –
   c. a person just before a meal than for a person just after a meal 10. –
   d. for a senior high-school girl than for a senior high-school boy of the same age and build............................... 11. –

4. In attempting to reduce one's weight:
   a. one should use the height-weight table as a general guide, but be more concerned about sudden changes in weight......... 12. +
   b. one should limit one's intake of sweets and pastries......... 13. +
   c. one should intelligently take in less calories each day than one uses.. 14. +
   d. one should limit one's diet to a few foods having low energy value... 15. –

5. The energy expended by the body can be measured:
   a. in terms of the oxygen used.............................. 16. +
   b. in terms of the carbon dioxide given out.................. 17. +
   c. in terms of calories—a food calorie being the amount of heat necessary to raise one kilogram of water one degree centigrade 18. +
   d. by a respiration apparatus................................ 19. +

6. Basal metabolism is:
   a. the amount of energy an individual needs when lying awake comfortably relaxed twelve to fourteen hours after the last meal.. 20. +
   b. 110 calories per hour for the average man................. 21. –

7. The energy need of an individual is calculated in terms of the calories needed for his basal metabolism, plus an additional amount for his other energy needs.................................. 22. +

8. The energy value of foods:
   a. can be determined by burning them in a bomb calorimeter and measuring the heat they give off........................... 23. +
   b. is frequently represented as "shares" of daily requirement, each share representing 1/30 of daily need of average man... 24. +
   c. is frequently represented as "shares," one energy share being 100 calories... 25. +
   d. is about 4 calories per gram of carbohydrate, 9 calories per gram of fat, and 4 calories per gram of protein............. 26. +

9. The digestion of:
   a. food is a process of changing food substances into a simple, soluble form.................................... 27. +
   b. starch takes place in the stomach and in the intestine....... 28. −
   c. protein takes place in the stomach and in the intestine...... 29. +

10. Digested foods are absorbed into the body from the alimentary canal:
   a. by the process of osmosis................................ 30. +
   b. chiefly from the stomach wall........................... 31. −
   c. into many capillaries and lacteals located in the wall of the digestive tract.. 32. +
   d. the absorptive surface being increased by minute fingerlike processes of the mucous membrane........................ 33. +

11. The body gets energy when carbondioxide combines with food in the cells of the body.................................... 34. −

12. For the body to get energy over a long period of time both food and oxygen must be distributed in cells throughout the body.... 35. +

13. The circulatory system—
   a. consists of a heart, blood, and vessels called arteries, veins, and capillaries.. 36. +
   b. distributes food and oxygen throughout the body and removes wastes from cells of the body.......................... 37. +
   c. sends blood through two sets of capillaries in that portion of the blood stream which absorbs food from the digestive tract before it returns to the heart........................... 38. +

14. The blood and lymph:
   a. serve as a fluid means of transportation for distribution of all raw materials to body cells and for removal of all waste products from them.................................... 39. +
   b. must be relatively stable in composition else sickness results... 40. +

15. The concentration of sugar in the blood is regulated by insulin... 41. +

16. It takes the following to furnish one energy "share":
   a. 4 squares of butter..................................... 42. −
   b. 2 tablespoonfuls granulated sugar....................... 43. +

17. These shares are found in the following quantities in foods:
   a. 1 to 3 shares each of calcium, phosphorus and iron in one egg 44. +
   b. 10 to 12 shares of calcium, 4 to 5 shares of phosphorus and less than one of iron in one ounce of American cheese........... 45. +

18. Other things besides energy which must be watched carefully in the American diet are to make sure that phosphorus, iron and calcium are present in sufficient amounts..................... 46. +

19. In selecting a diet one should consider protective or regulative foods in the following ways:
    a. one must be sure to have a sufficient supply to furnish the essentials without which the body cannot function............ 47. +
    b. it is desirable to maintain wide margins of these foods...... 48. +
    c. vitamins A, B, and C can be taken in large amounts, but one should be cautious about vitamin D..................... 49. −
    d. care must be taken not to get too much of these protective foods because of their harmful effects when taken in large quantities.................................... 50. −

20. Vitamin A:
    a. is a relatively close derivative of carotene and hence is found in yellow vegetables and fruits.......................... 51. +
    b. in one ounce, a small serving, of carrots is 15 shares......... 52. +

21. Vitamin B:
    a. is needed by the body for normal appetite, digestion and assimilation of food, and to prevent beriberi .... 53. +
    b. is abundantly supplied in most highly refined foods......... 54. −
    c. is found abundantly in yeast and in wheat embryo.......... 55. +
    d. content of the average American diet is deficient............ 56. +

22. Vitamin C:
    a. is added to a number of the foods one buys as a concentrate or by irradiation.................................... 57. −
    b. is used to advantage by the body in amounts well over minimal need.. 58. +
    c. in one small glass of orange or tomato juice is 50 shares..... 59. +
    d. is the most stable of the vitamins........................ 60. −

23. Vitamin D:
    a. is necessary for calcium and phosphorus assimilation........ 61. +
    b. is dangerous in concentrated form........................ 62. −
    c. is mainly supplied by fish oils, egg yolk, and milk........... 63. +
    d. is added to some of the foods one buys as a concentrate or by irradiation.................................... 64. +

24. Vitamins G and H:
    a. are essential to growth, nutrition and vitality.............. 65. +
    b. are abundantly found in eggs, liver, lean meats, vegetables and fruits.. 66. +
    c. are dangerous in amounts above normal need.............. 67. −
    d. are advantageous in amounts considerably above normal need 68. +

25. So-called "whole" foods:
    a. are safer than refined foods from the standpoint of getting rich supplies of the protective and regulative foods.............. 69. +

b. include whole wheat cereal, unpolished rice, rolled oats, fresh fruits, oysters, and clams.............................. 70. +

26. Foods may be classified according to their usefulness to us:
   a. milk, white rice, olives, and eggs are considered protective foods.. 71. −
   b. cereals, potatoes, rice, sweets, and fats are outstanding energy-producing foods.................................. 72. +

27. Vitamins can be saved by following such rules in cookery as:
   a. thoroughly cook all vegetables......................... 73. −
   b. use lots of water when cooking vegetables.................. 74. −

28. Application of one's knowledge of foods may be made by:
   a. seeing that the vitamins in foods are not lost by cooking..... 75. +
   b. selecting half of one's energy shares from protective foods.... 76. +

29. The newer knowledge of nutrition indicates that one may reasonably expect:
   a. to insure one's vigor, alertness and energy by proper selection of foods.. 77. +
   b. to mature more rapidly, live more vigorously, and postpone old age appreciably.................................. 78. +

CONSTRUCTING THE ADVERTISEMENT INTERPRETATION TEST

The judging of the truthfulness of current food advertisements offered an opportunity to test the pupil's use of knowledge in rating them. Many of these statements have a scientific background, but are so related to other elements that they tend to create an erroneous impression.

Seventy-one verbatim statements were copied from fifteen food advertisements found in current magazines. These items were arranged in a trial form. The test was then given to a group of 30 pupils who were asked to rate the items on a five-point scale ranging from wholly false to wholly true. This scale was later abandoned for a four-point scale because it proved quite impossible to judge the degree of truthfulness or falsity on so fine a scale.

A group of nutrition students and home economics teachers checked the scale. Their combined judgments were used in scoring the test in its trial form.

The scores made by the trial group were arranged in descending order, and the upper quartile and the lower quartile were determined. Then the number of correct responses made by the upper quartile on each item was determined. The same was done for the lower quartile. Those items were discarded which failed to distinguish between the upper quartile and the lower quartile.

Several evaluation experts[10] critically examined the test. Ambiguous items were discarded. Compound items were divided to make simpler ones. The test was then put in its final form. This form was used throughout the first experiment and the extended experiment.

To further guarantee that the rating of this test, Test No. 3, "Advertisement Interpretation Test," was in agreement with the opinions of experts in the field, the same group of twenty advanced nutrition students who checked the other two tests also checked this one. Points of credit were given to responses in terms of the tendency of the experts to agree in checking.

No. of Judges Agreeing on a Response	Points Assigned to Responses
18-20	5
15-17	4
13-14	3
9-12	2
8	1

The cumulative points assigned to responses gave a scale of eighty-six points of credit on twenty-eight items.

The test was then divided into paired halves to determine its reliability,[11] as indicated below:

	One Half	Other Half
Number of test items	14	14
Number of responses credited	15	16
Number of "A" responses credited	1	1
Number of "B" responses credited	1	1
Number of "C" responses credited	2	2
Number of "D" responses credited	11	12
Points of credit assigned	43	43

The final form of the test "Advertisement Interpretation Test," is given in the following pages.

[10] Six members of the staff of the Commission on Evaluation in the Eight Year Study, Progressive Education Association.

[11] Cf. page 84.

Test No. 3. "Advertisement Interpretation Test"

Directions. Following are statements taken from several advertisements. They express varying degrees of truthfulness. In some cases a part truth is stated in such a way as to be misleading to the reader. In other cases undue emphasis tends to give the reader a false impression. Place a check in the column which you believe best rates the truthfulness of the statements given.

Key to the Columns

Column A. . . . . Wholly false.
Column B. . . . . Improbable, unlikely to be true.
Column C. . . . . Probable, likely to be true.
Column D. . . . . Wholly true.

	A	B	C	D
I. Refined Milled Products Advertisement				
1. Diet and health are intimately bound together. . . .				5*
2. Bread is our outstanding source of the largest single need in the balanced diet—food energy.				3
3. Bread is a most economical source of food energy				3
4. There is almost no waste in white bread as it is 96% digested.				2
5. The control of weight depends solely on the food-energy content of the diet as a whole, not on any one specific food in the diet.				3
II. Rolled Oats Advertisement				
6. [Nervousness, constipation and poor appetite] prey on the energy of thousands, young and old, because their diets do not contain enough of the precious vitamin B.			1	2
7. Rolled oats supplies plenty of vitamin B to combat nervousness, constipation, and poor appetite due to lack of vitamin B.			2	
III. Cheese Advertisements				
8. To cut costs without sacrificing food value, give a [cheese] dish the stellar role on your menu.			2	2
9. These famous cheeses supply nutrition richly concentrated.			2	
10. [These cheeses supply] vitamin A—plus a wealth of the precious milk minerals including calcium and phosphorus.				4
IV. Dessert Advertisement				
11. Dextrose is a sugar, the normal sugar of the human body.				3
12. Dextrose is instantly digested; in fact it is immediately absorbed by the bloodstream.				2
13. Dextrose requires no digestive effort.				1

* Points of credit assigned.

	A	B	C	D
V. Oleomargarine Advertisement				
14. [Oleomargarine is] perfect for baking—on vegetables—for making gravies and sauces, and for frying		1		
15. Oleomargarine is fine for growing children	3	1		
VI. Canned Goods Advertisements				
16. Canned foods rank among the best food we eat	1			
17. Canned salmon helps in creating better balanced meals because it brings us so many essential food values				1
18. Salmon is a rich source of protein, the food factor that builds up our tissues				4
19. [Canned salmon] also gives us phosphorus, and the great goitre-preventative, iodine				3
VII. Cod Liver Oil Advertisement				
20. Bad weather, clothing, even smoke and clouds, shut out the protective "vitamin D" rays except for a relatively few days of the year				3
21. Indoors, ordinary window glass prevents the sun's rays from being effective				4
22. A good cod liver oil provides an abundance, not only of vitamin D, but also of vitamin A				5
23. Babies need vitamin A to build general resistance and to help them grow				5
24. The way to judge the cost of cod liver oil is by the number of vitamin units it contains, not by the size or price of the bottle				4
VIII. Yeast Advertisement				
25. If you take laxatives to keep "regular," you know from experience that drugs and cathartics give only temporary relief from constipation				5
26. Doctors now know that in many cases the real cause of constipation is a shortage of vitamin B				3
27. [Fresh yeast] steps up the activity of the digestive organs				2
28. Yeast is the richest known food source of vitamins B and G				4

The coefficients of correlations for the three tests—Attitudes, Information, and Applications of Principles—follow in Table I.

TABLE I

THE RELIABILITY OF THE TESTS

Groups in School B	N	r_{xy}	r_{2II}	Levels of Significance*	
				1%	5%
		Test 1 (Attitudes)			
A.	24	.542	.704	.515	.404
B.	26	.475	.646	.496	.388
C.	29	.752	.859	.470	.367
ABC.	79	.677	.806	.293	.225
		Test 2 (Information)			
A.	24	.491	.658	.515	.404
B.	26	.629	.722	.496	.388
C.	29	.376	.540	.470	.367
ABC.	79	.599	.749	.293	.225
		Test 3 (Applications)			
A.	24	.802	.890	.515	.404
B.	26	.524	.621	.496	.388
C.	27	.586	.739	.470	.367
ABC.	79	.606	.754	.293	.225

r_{xy} = correlation between halves. r_{2II} = Spearman-Brown correction.

* Fisher's test of significance has been applied to the correlations obtained. This gives the probability that a correlation as large as the one obtained could arise by random sampling from an uncorrelated population. By "significant" is meant that there are five chances in 100 that the coefficient will arise from an uncorrelated population (i.e., the chance is .05). By "very significant" is meant a similar probability that the coefficient will appear in one chance out of 100 or less. Fisher, R. A., *Statistical Methods for Research Workers*, Oliver and Boyd, Edinburgh, 1937.

We may consider the reliability coefficient of each test that obtained from the total group after applying the Spearman-Brown correction. Thus the reliability of the attitudes test is .806, that of the information test .749, and that of the applications test .754.

CHAPTER V

Data of the Experiment

THE problem of this study is, "Can the study of the relation of food to physical well-being be truly educative?" That is, are the outcomes of instruction such that boys and girls use it in their daily lives? Do they select their diets more wisely after having had such instruction? Do they increasingly reorganize their judgments and habits concerning nutrition in the light of new data? Objective evidence on this problem is gained from an analysis of the scores obtained on the attitudes, information, and applications of principles tests, and from careful scrutiny of the anecdotes. The first part of this chapter gives the data obtained from the use of the tests; the second part gives descriptions of pupil behavior in the study of nutrition along with an appraisal of the organization of the materials by the participating teachers.

THE RESULTS OF THE FIRST EXPERIMENT

1. *Do the data show that the experimental group made significant gains in each of the attributes measured?*

Table II gives the means on the initial and final tests (Tests 1, 2, and 3) for all pupils participating in the experiment. There is a considerable increase in each final mean over each initial mean. This increase is very marked in Test 2, "Information." The gains, together with their variability, are presented in Table III. Table IV shows that the gains made in the final test over the initial test may all be considered significant.

That these gains are due to the experimental factor is shown by the data presented in Tables V, VI, VII, and VIII. Table V shows the bases used in matching the control and the experimental groups. Table VI gives the means of the scores made on the initial, final, and retention tests. Table VII shows the mean of the gains made in the final tests and the retention tests over the intial tests, together with the variability of those gains. Table VIII gives the means of the gains and their significance.

The control group shown in Table V was secured by giving the initial and final tests to a class of pupils not studying nutrition. From this control class it was possible to match a group of fifteen pupils against a similar group of fifteen pupils in the experimental class. This matching was done on the basis of age, intelligence quotient, and initial test scores on Tests 1, 2, and 3. The groups were equated by making a distribution of the position of all of the members of the experimental and control groups in each of the bases used in matching. Then those individuals which destroyed the similarity of the mean and variability of each distribution were "peeled off." This was done by eliminating the cases within the step interval where the number was greatest. By this process five pairs of distributions were made having similar frequencies in each step interval. Table V shows how closely the means and variability of the two groups compared.

Table VI gives an opportunity to compare the means made on each of the final tests by the experimental and the control groups. The difference in favor of the experimental group indicates that the experimental factor caused the shift. In fact, the control group lost in two of the three tests.

Table VII shows clearly the gains made in the final tests over the initial tests by the experimental group. Table VIII shows that all the gains made by the experimental group are highly significant. At the same time, the control group lost on two of the tests and failed to make a significant gain on the third one.

The data for both the entire experimental group and for the smaller matched group show that the pupils made significant gains in each of the three attributes measured.

2. *Do the data show that the experimental group retained a significant portion of the gains made in each attribute one year after the classroom work on nutrition?*

Table II gives the means on both the retention tests and the initial tests. The former are all higher than the latter. Table III shows the gains made on the retention tests over the initial tests and the final tests. These data indicate that when we consider the results for all of the individuals in the experimental groups, they retain practically

TABLE II

MEANS OF SCORES MADE BY ALL PUPILS IN THE EXPERIMENTAL GROUP AT LINCOLN SCHOOL, WHO COMPLETED EACH INITIAL, FINAL, AND RETENTION TEST, 1936-37[1]

Test	*N*	M_I	M_F	M_R
1—Attitudes..........	32	30.03	36.03	35.75
2—Information.......	28	23.43	40.68	33.25
3—Applications.......	34	30.94	38.09	33.35

[1] The initial and final tests were given during the spring of 1936. The retention test was given during the spring of 1937.

all of their gain in attitude, approximately two-thirds of their gain in information, and approximately one-third of their ability to apply this knowledge in the interpretation of advertisements. Table IV shows that they retain a significant portion of their gain in attitude and information.

The results obtained from the matched groups (Tables VI, VII, and VIII) show that the experimental group actually made a gain in the retention tests over the final tests in attitude and in application of principles in the interpretation of advertising material. This increase, however, is not significantly high, so it is more accurate to

TABLE III

GAINS MADE BY ALL PUPILS IN THE EXPERIMENTAL GROUP AT LINCOLN SCHOOL, WHO COMPLETED EACH INITIAL, FINAL, AND RETENTION TEST, 1936-37

Test	*N*	Gains in Final Over Initial Tests		Gains in Retention Over Initial Tests		Gains in Retention Over Final Tests
		$\overline{G}_{I\text{-}F}$*	σ_G	$\overline{G}_{I\text{-}R}$	σ_G	$\overline{G}_{F\text{-}R}$
1—Attitudes.......	32	6.00	13.31	5.72	13.96	−0.28
2—Information....	28	17.25	12.29	9.82	12.66	−7.43
3—Applications....	34	7.15	13.27	2.41	17.31	−4.74

* Mean gain, $\overline{G}_{I\text{-}F}$, was computed by the formula $\overline{G}_{I\text{-}F} = \frac{\Sigma + \text{'s} - \Sigma - \text{'s}}{N}$. Standard deviation, σ_G, was computed by the formula $\sigma_G = \sqrt{\frac{\Sigma G^2}{N} - \overline{G}^2}$, where $\overline{G}^2$ represents the square of the difference made by each pupil on the initial and final tests.

TABLE IV

SIGNIFICANCE OF GAINS MADE BY ALL PUPILS IN THE EXPERIMENTAL GROUP AT LINCOLN SCHOOL, WHO COMPLETED EACH INITIAL, FINAL, AND RETENTION TEST, 1936-37

		Gains in Final Over Initial Tests			Gains in Retention Over Initial Tests		
Test	*N*	$\overline{G}_{I-F}$*	$\sigma_{\overline{G}}$*	$\overline{G}/\sigma_{\overline{G}}$*	$\overline{G}_{I-R}$	σ_G	$\overline{G}/\sigma_{\overline{G}}$
1—Attitudes.......	32	6.00	2.35	2.54	5.72	2.47	2.31
2—Information....	28	17.25	2.32	7.44	9.82	2.39	4.10
3—Applications....	34	7.15	2.28	3.10	2.41	2.97	0.82

* $\overline{G}$ = mean gain; $\sigma_{\overline{G}}$ = standard error; $\overline{G}/\sigma_{\overline{G}}$ = ratio mean gain to standard error.

TABLE V

BASES USED IN MATCHING GROUPS AT LINCOLN SCHOOL, 1936

		Means									
Group	*N*	Age[1]		I.Q.[2]		Test 1		Test 2		Test 3	
		M	$\sigma_{Dist.}$	M	$\sigma_{Dist.}$	M	$\sigma_{Dist.}$	M	$\sigma_{Dist.}$	M	$\sigma_{Dist.}$
Experimental.......	15	14-10.3	9.1	124.9	9.5	26.4	1.9	25.2	3.0	28.4	4.6
Control............	15	14- 6.9	9.3	120.0	12.3	29.2	1.5	25.0	3.1	24.8	5.1
Difference in means of two groups.......		+3.4		+4.9		−2.8		+0.2		+3.6	

[1] Age is given in years and months as of April, 1936.
[2] Intelligence Quotient was obtained with Stanford Binet Test.

TABLE VI

MEANS OF SCORES MADE ON INITIAL, FINAL, AND RETENTION TESTS BY MATCHED EXPERIMENTAL AND CONTROL GROUP AT LINCOLN SCHOOL, 1936-37*

Test	Group	*N*	M_I	M_F	M_R
1—Attitudes	Experimental..............	15	26.40	38.80	39.69
	Control....................	15	29.21	23.41	23.28
2—Information	Experimental..............	15	25.20	38.20	34.53
	Control....................	15	25.00	17.87	16.73
3—Applications	Experimental..............	15	28.40	40.00	41.20
	Control....................	15	24.80	27.47	24.13

* Initial and final tests were given during the spring of 1936; retention test during the spring of 1937.

TABLE VII

GAINS MADE IN FINAL AND RETENTION OVER INITIAL TESTS BY MATCHED EXPERIMENTAL AND CONTROL GROUP AT LINCOLN SCHOOL, 1936-37

Test	Group	N	Gains in Final Over Initial Tests $\bar{G}_{I-F}$	σ_G	Gains in Retention Over Initial Tests $\bar{G}_{I-R}$	σ_G	Gains in Retention Over Final Tests $\bar{G}_{F-R}$
1—Attitudes	Experimental...	15	12.40	14.66	13.27	11.25	0.87
	Control........	15	−5.80	13.73	−5.93	12.01	−0.13
2—Information	Experimental...	15	13.00	9.76	9.33	12.68	−3.67
	Control........	15	−7.13	8.29	−8.27	6.97	−1.14
3—Applications	Experimental...	15	11.60	12.45	12.80	15.02	1.20
	Control........	15	2.67	13.69	−0.67	11.49	−3.34

say that they retained all the gains made in these two attributes a year after instruction. They retained approximately three-fourths of the gains made in information.

The variation between the results obtained with the matched groups and the results obtained with the experimental groups can be accounted for by the fact that matching on five bases tends somewhat to destroy the randomness of the sample. When the tedium of taking tests for the third time is considered, as shown by the losses of the control group, one may say with certainty that the gains on the Retention test over Initial Tests 1 and 2 are significant, and

TABLE VIII

SIGNIFICANCE OF GAINS MADE IN FINAL AND RETENTION TESTS OVER INITIAL TESTS BY MATCHED EXPERIMENTAL AND CONTROL GROUP AT LINCOLN SCHOOL, 1936-37

Test	Group	N	Gains in Final Over Initial Tests $\bar{G}$	$\sigma_{\bar{G}}$	$\bar{G}/\sigma_{\bar{G}}$	Gains in Retention Over Initial Tests $\bar{G}$	$\sigma_{\bar{G}}$	$\bar{G}/\sigma_{\bar{G}}$
1—Attitudes	Experimental..	15	12.40	3.78	3.28	13.27	2.90	4.57
	Control.......	15	−5.80	3.54	(1.67)	−5.93	3.10	(1.87)
2—Information	Experimental..	15	13.00	2.52	5.16	9.33	3.25	2.87
	Control.......	15	−7.13	2.14	(3.33)	−8.27	1.77	(4.67)
3—Applications	Experimental..	15	11.60	3.21	3.61	12.80	3.88	3.30
	Control.......	15	2.67	3.77	0.71	−0.67	2.99	(0.02)

may state with considerable conviction that those made on Test 3 are also significant.

Summary. The experimental group made significant gains in each attribute measured.

The experimental group retained a significant portion of the gains made in each attribute.

The gains could not be attributed to the practice effect of taking the tests.

The gains are in all probability due to the experimental factor.

THE RESULTS OF THE EXTENDED EXPERIMENT

1. *Do the data show that the experimental groups in the various school systems made significant gains in their attitude toward the selection of diet?*

TABLE IX

MEAN OF SCORES MADE BY ALL PUPILS WHO PARTICIPATED IN THE EXTENDED EXPERIMENT AND WHO COMPLETED EACH INITIAL AND FINAL TEST, 1937

Group	*N*	Attitudes-Test 1		Information-Test 2		Applications-Test 3	
		M_I	M_F	M_I	M_F	M_I	M_F
Lincoln Biology	17	46.70	59.53	26.35	42.47	31.41	39.41
Lincoln 9th Grade	46	53.70	65.66	19.41	48.45	31.15	41.43
School H	27	67.96	79.46	37.33	48.37	40.11	49.70
School B	79	60.54	74.04	16.53	37.53	36.21	42.58
School E	15	63.67	74.87	32.60	41.87	37.00	38.07
School C	18	60.61	81.17	14.83	54.94	32.22	40.72
School G	56	81.10	88.67	11.21	29.10	34.38	41.38
School D Teacher 1	44	27.57	31.25	20.95	29.06	34.25	33.64
School D Teacher 2	46	27.69	25.71	18.42	21.96	31.87	33.28
School A Teacher 1	76	25.87	26.15	18.34	21.68	....	....
School A Teacher 2	27	30.52	34.08	19.78	25.82	....	....
School I Control							
Test 1	46	50.84	49.49				
Test 2	42			26.71	27.35		
Test 3	31					33.10	39.74

Table IX shows that when we compare the means of the scores which all pupils in the various experimental groups made on initial and final tests, nine out of the eleven final means are considerably above the initial means. Table X gives the mean gains and their variability of each of the groups. Table XI shows that nine of the eleven mean gains in attitude may be considered significant. At the same time those pupils in School I who took the tests without the experimental work showed a mean loss.

As in the first experiment,[2] groups were matched with a control group in order to be sure that changes observed were due to the experimental factor. The descriptions of the locations of Schools B, C, G, and I[3] indicate that the socio-economic status of individuals from these localities would be quite comparable. Therefore it should be possible to rely upon results obtained by matching groups of pupils in these situations. Table XII shows the bases used in matching. A group of 30 pupils from School B were matched against a group of 15 pupils from School I on age and initial test scores on Tests 1, 2, and 3. A group of 15 pupils from School C were matched against 15 pupils from School I on age, intelligence quotients, and initial test scores on Tests 1, 2, and 3. A group of 15 home economics pupils from School G were matched against the same control

TABLE X

GAINS MADE BY ALL PUPILS WHO PARTICIPATED IN THE EXTENDED EXPERIMENT AND WHO COMPLETED EACH INITIAL AND FINAL TEST, 1937

Group	N	Attitudes-Test 1		Information-Test 2		Applications-Test 3	
		$\overline{G}$	σ_G	$\overline{G}$	σ_G	$\overline{G}$	σ_G
Lincoln Biology	17	12.83	15.50	16.12	14.58	8.00	15.62
Lincoln 9th Grade	46	11.96	18.17	29.04	10.18	10.28	13.68
School H	27	11.50	18.06	11.04	9.54	9.59	13.25
School B	79	13.50	17.09	21.00	11.90	6.37	15.28
School E	15	11.20	11.37	9.27	6.87	1.07	16.26
School C	18	20.56	16.97	40.11	9.80	8.50	9.06
School G	56	7.57	17.85	17.89	13.33	7.00	13.53
School D Teacher 1	44	3.68	10.74	8.11	10.91	−0.61	19.65
School D Teacher 2	46	−1.98	11.27	3.54	11.67	1.41	13.49
School A Teacher 1	76	0.28	10.50	3.34	13.73	....	....
School A Teacher 2	27	3.56	8.45	6.04	11.38	....	....
School I Control							
Test 1	46	−1.35	15.49				
Test 2	42			0.64	12.63		
Test 3	31					6.64	14.64

[2] Cf. page 9.

[3] Cf. page 12.

TABLE XI

SIGNIFICANCE OF GAINS MADE BY ALL PUPILS WHO PARTICIPATED IN THE EXTENDED EXPERIMENT AND WHO COMPLETED EACH INITIAL AND FINAL TEST, 1937

Group	N	Attitudes-Test 1			Information-Test 2			Applications-Test 3		
		$\overline{G}$	$\sigma_{\overline{G}}$	$\overline{G}/\sigma_{\overline{G}}$	$\overline{G}$	$\sigma_{\overline{G}}$	$\overline{G}/\sigma_{\overline{G}}$	$\overline{G}$	$\sigma_{\overline{G}}$	$\overline{G}/\sigma_{\overline{G}}$
Lincoln Biology	17	12.83	3.76	3.4	16.12	3.54	4.6	8.00	3.79	2.1
Lincoln 9th Grade...	46	11.96	2.68	4.1	29.04	1.50	19.4	10.28	2.02	5.1
School H......	27	11.50	3.54	3.2	11.04	1.83	6.0	9.59	2.54	3.8
School B......	79	13.50	1.90	7.1	21.00	1.35	15.7	6.37	1.72	3.7
School E......	15	11.20	2.94	3.8	9.27	1.78	5.2	1.07	4.20	0.3
School C......	18	20.56	3.06	6.7	40.11	2.31	17.3	8.50	2.14	4.0
School G......	56	7.57	2.38	3.2	17.89	1.78	10.0	7.00	1.86	3.7
School D Teacher 1...	44	3.68	1.62	2.3	8.11	1.64	4.9	−0.61	2.96	(0.2)
School D Teacher 2...	46	−1.98	1.66	(1.2)	3.54	1.72	2.1	1.41	1.99	.08
School A Teacher 1...	76	0.28	1.21	0.2	3.34	1.57	2.1	....	...	...
School A Teacher 2...	27	3.56	1.63	2.2	6.04	2.19	2.8	....	...	...
School I Control										
Test 1......	46	−1.35	2.28	(0.6)						
Test 2......	42				0.64	1.95	0.3			
Test 3......	31							6.64	2.63	2.5

* Reliability of mean gain; a ratio of 3 is considered virtual certainty; Garrett, op. cit., those ratios above which are less than 3 represent the following chances in 100 that the true difference is greater than zero:

Ratio....................	.2	.3	.6	.8	1.2	2.1	2.2	2.3	2.5	2.8
Chances in 100............	58.	62.	73.	79.	88.	98.	98.6	98.9	99.4	99.7

TABLE XII

BASES USED IN MATCHING GROUPS IN THE EXTENDED EXPERIMENT, 1937

Group	N	Age[1]		I.Q.[2]		Test 1[3]		Test 2		Test 3	
		M	$\sigma_{Dist.}$	M	$\sigma_{Dist.}$	M	$\sigma_{Dist.}$	M	$\sigma_{Dist.}$	M	$\sigma_{Dist.}$
School B.....	30	15-9.4	8.3			57.50	9.74	19.60	2.61	35.00	5.85
School C.....	15	15-5.0	6.3	111.3	15.5	61.80	14.42	17.21	2.96	33.60	5.14
School G.....	15	15-1.7	5.9	113.1	17.3	66.32	5.99	19.2	3.21	22.60	3.18
School I Control......	15	15-8.5		113.1		57.40		21.59		36.40	

[1] Age is given in years and months as of April, 1937.

[2] Intelligent Quotient obtained in Schools C and I from Henman-Nelson A and in School G from the Otis Self-Administering Test; quotients were not available for School B.

[3] School G was not equated on Test 1.

TABLE XIII

GAINS MADE IN FINAL TESTS OVER INITIAL TESTS BY MATCHED GROUPS IN THE EXTENDED EXPERIMENT, 1937

Group	N	Attitudes-Test 1		Information-Test 2		Applications-Test 3	
		$\overline{G}_{I-F}$	σ_G	$\overline{G}_{I-F}$	σ_G	$\overline{G}_{I-F}$	σ_G
School B.	30	16.80	16.49	20.73	23.24	6.83	15.58
School C.	15	21.67	16.37	40.40	9.90	7.67	11.68
School G.	15	12.40	10.89	14.13	11.13	6.00	9.66
School I Control.	15	3.27	15.72	2.07	10.43	0.80	14.56

group from School I on age, intelligence quotients, and initial test scores on Tests 2 and 3. It was impossible to match this latter group on the initial test score of Test 1.

Table XIII shows that the gain made on Test 1 by each matched experimental group is much greater than that made by the control group. Table XIV shows that each experimental group made highly significant gains, while those made by the control group were not significant. The gains must be due to the experimental factor.

2. *Do the data show that the experimental groups in the various schools made significant gains in nutrition information?*

Tables IX, X, and XI show that all of the experimental groups made significantly high gains in information, whereas the control group made practically no gain. Four of the eleven groups made an unbelievably high gain. The two groups making the least significant gains in information were the same as those not making significant gains in attitude. School D had over 90 pupils and School A over 103 pupils taking the work. In both of these schools library facilities were limited. While each school had two sets of the most essential reference books listed in the unit suitable study materials were not available in the textbooks. When one considers how difficult it would be for the many pupils in these schools to have access to any reference material, it seems quite remarkable that they made the gains shown. Teacher 2 in School D wrote that the pupils found the vocabulary of the tests difficult. Probably some of this difficulty was due to lack of reading material.

A study of the matched groups in Tables XIII and XIV shows

TABLE XIV

SIGNIFICANCE OF GAINS MADE IN FINAL TESTS OVER INITIAL TESTS BY MATCHED GROUPS IN THE EXTENDED EXPERIMENT, 1937

Group	N	Attitudes-Test 1			Information-Test 2			Applications-Test 3		
		$\bar{G}$	$\sigma_{\bar{G}}$	$\bar{G}/\sigma_{\bar{G}}$*	$\bar{G}$	$\sigma_{\bar{G}}$	$\bar{G}/\sigma_{\bar{G}}$	$\bar{G}$	$\sigma_{\bar{G}}$	$\bar{G}/\sigma_{\bar{G}}$
School B......	30	16.80	3.01	5.58	20.73	4.24	4.89	6.83	2.84	2.43
School C......	15	21.67	4.22	5.12	40.40	2.56	15.79	7.67	3.02	2.79
School G......	15	12.40	2.24	5.54	14.13	2.87	4.91	6.00	2.49	2.41
School I Control	15	3.27	4.06	0.80	2.07	2.69	0.76	0.80	3.76	0.21

* Reliability of mean gain; a ratio of 3 is considered virtual certainty; Garrett, *op. cit.:* those ratios above which are less than 3 represent the following chances in 100 that the true difference is greater than zero:

Ratio....................	0.2	0.8	2.4	2.8
Chances in 100...........	58.	79.	99.2	99.7

that the experimental groups all made very significant gains in Test 2, whereas the control group did not make appreciable gains. Hence the changes observed must have been due to the experimental factor.

3. *Do the data show that the experimental groups in the various schools made significant gains in the application of nutrition principles?*

Tables IX, X, and XI show that six of the nine experimental groups made gains which may be considered significant. There is no evidence from School A, as the initial tests were not given there. Two of the experimental groups not making significant gains were from School D, where the gains in knowledge had been relatively low. School E failed to show significant gains in the use of knowledge. This may be due to lack of contact with current food advertisements in the small rural community where School E is located. It may also be due to slight emphasis on the *use* of knowledge in classroom procedures. Surprisingly enough, the control group made gains which may be considered significant. Investigation revealed that the control biology group had been doing some work in consumer education during the interim between the tests. It seems logical to attribute their gain to such instruction rather than to a practice effect in the taking of the tests. The control group in the first experiment, which was given at Lincoln School, showed no such gains, hence there is little reason to believe a practice effect enters into the scores made.

When the gains made by the matched groups are considered, as shown in Tables XIII and XIV, all experimental groups made gains which may be considered significant, while the control group did not make significant gains.

Summary. Nine of the eleven experimental groups in the various schools made significant gains on Test 1. The two schools not making significant gains did not have adequate reference material.

All experimental groups in the various schools showed significant gains on Test 2.

Six of the nine experimental groups showed significant gains on Test 3. Two of those not showing such gains were from schools handicapped for reference material.

All of the matched experimental groups made significant gains in each attribute measured.

The gains observed in the scores made by the experimental groups were due to the experimental factor.

Some groups gained relatively more on Test 1 than others, some more on Test 2 than others, and some more on Test 3 than others. This can be partially explained by the fact that each teacher would give a slightly different emphasis to his teaching.

THE EVIDENCE FROM THE INTERCORRELATIONS BETWEEN THE SCORES MADE ON THE TESTS

1. *Do the intercorrelations show that Tests 1, 2, and 3 each measure separate attributes?*

Of the sixty intercorrelations given in Table XV there are but eight which may be considered significantly above zero; of those eight there are but two which may be considered highly significant. Five are negative. Hence the tests surely measure different attributes.

2. *How do the intercorrelations made between the initial tests compare with those made between the final tests?*

Six of the nine intercorrelations between Tests 1 and 2 are higher for the initial tests than for the final tests; six of the nine intercorrelations between Tests 2 and 3 are higher for the initial tests; six of the nine intercorrelations between Tests 1 and 3 are higher for the initial tests. In other words, eighteen of the twenty-seven intercorrelations between the scores made by the experimental groups were higher when the pupils began their study than when they finished it.

If only those intercorrelations which are significantly above zero are considered, six of the eight are found between the initial test scores. The two which may be considered highly significant are both between initial test scores.

Thus the intercorrelations between the final tests are lower than those between the initial tests. This is quite surprising since practically all experimental groups made gains on each final test over each initial test. In other words, it is not safe to assume that a high intercorrelation exists between two tests when a given group shows significant gains in both of them.

TABLE XV

INTERCORRELATIONS BETWEEN SCORES MADE ON TESTS 1, 2, AND 3

	Initial Test			Final Test			N	Significance Level (Fisher's Table)	
	r_{I-II}	r_{II-III}	r_{I-III}	r_{I-II}	r_{II-III}	r_{I-III}		5%	1%
Lincoln Biology	.050	.246	−.025	.199	.539	.334	17	.482	.606
Lincoln 9th Grade	.386	.256	−.024	.154	.153	.364	46	.291	.376
School H	.191	.239	.351	.237	.233	.019	26	.388	.496
School B	.149	.215	.238	.061	.161	.174	79	.225	.293
School E	.479	.610	.465	.433	.031	.368	15	.514	.641
School C	.411	.396	.510	.431	.102	.145	18	.468	.590
School G	.039	.039	.209	−.143	.089	.160	48	.285	.369
School D Teacher 1	.439	.144	.481	.115	−.109	.265	44	.298	.384
School D Teacher 2	.270	.215	−.0076	.066	.234	.229	46	.291	.576
School I Control	.241	.175	−.063	−.129	.296	.110	28	.374	.478

r_{I-II} = Correlation between Test 1 and Test 2.
r_{II-III} = Correlation between Test 2 and Test 3.
r_{I-III} = Correlation between Test 1 and Test 3.

Significance Level: r below 5% level may be considered not significant; r between 5% and 1% may be considered significant; r above 1% may be considered highly significant.

Even though the organization of the materials was supposedly such as to foster an integration of experiences related to nutrition, pupils did not progress in integration of experiences toward the goal held by the experts. Some pupils apparently made large gains in attitude and little in information or use of information; others made large gains in information and little in attitude or use of information; and still others made large gains in use of information but little in attitude or information.

3. *How do we account for the lowering of the intercorrelations on the final tests?*

Pupil interest may partially account for this trend toward lower intercorrelations between the related though separate attributes. Methods of teaching apparently account for some of the trend. In the Lincoln School four of the six higher intercorrelations were found between the final tests. Teacher 2 in School D also had two of his three higher intercorrelations between final tests. Three of the remaining groups had two of the three higher intercorrelations between initial tests. The other three groups had all three of the higher intercorrelations between the initial tests. The fact that pupils vary in maturity may account for their failure to make an integration of experiences like that held desirable by experts.

4. *What evidence do those lowered intercorrelations throw upon the educative process?*

It is not safe to assume that pupils are making integrations of experiences similar to those of more mature persons even though they show gains on separate tests.

An organization which provides wide variety of pupil choice in the selection of experiences offers opportunity for pupils to grow in many ways. It is difficult to consider all the factors which affect a pupil's desire and ability to progress in any specific aspect.

The fact that it is possible to gain in any one attribute without gaining in the others may make it desirable to develop some attitudes or habits of action, and then as pupils mature, to provide those experiences which will enable them increasingly to use knowledge as a basis for intelligent action. Such a policy would demand much knowledge as to the maturity levels necessary for adequately grasping given fundamental concepts. This would also involve an increased understanding of the difficulties encountered in the mastery of these concepts.

It would seem highly desirable to investigate different methods of teaching to see the relation of such methods to the tendency of pupils to integrate the various aspects of given experiences.

The lowered intercorrelations bear witness to the fact that learning is a complex and difficult process, and that years of living with related problems are necessary to achieve an adult or expert understanding of the various factors related to any given concept.

Summary. The low intercorrelations between the tests indicate that each measures a separate attribute.

The lower intercorrelations between the final tests than between the initial tests indicate that the pupils progressed along divergent lines rather than achieving an integrated whole from the experience. It is evident that they must have many more contacts with the field to achieve mature understandings.

OTHER MEANS OF EVALUATING THE EXPERIMENT

Records of Pupil Behavior. Paper and pencil tests, no matter how numerous or how varied, do not give an adequate picture of pupil behavior. So the investigator has used other means of gathering evidence of how boys and girls use knowledge and apply principles they have learned to situations outside the classroom. The following records were taken from parents' written comments of pupil reactions in the home, stenographic reports of classroom work, and informal conversations with pupils.

One mother reports as follows:

I have noticed a decided change in John since he began his work in diet. I myself have been intensely interested in dietetics for years, but the changes I wanted to introduce in the home were received so belligerently that I was balked. John would not listen to any talk about vitamins: he refused whole wheat bread, insisted that white rice tasted much better than brown, etc. Now I hear him saying when he has his milk at bedtime, "I think I'll have an extra glass because I missed one today," or to his younger brother who is still protesting, "Cut it, you ought to be glad to get brown rice instead of polished rice."

He seems to be very much interested in calorie intake. I have heard him say, "I think I'll have something with my milk tonight (bedtime) just to make sure I have had all my calories." He stopped eating cereal at breakfast because he can't take milk after it and he thinks the milk is more important. When I discovered the reason, he agreed to take a small portion instead of the huge helping he had been taking, and he could still have the milk.

His former resistance is completely gone. I think the course has been most helpful and I am really grateful for the assistance that was given to me in my struggle to give my family the proper food.

Another parent notes that:

As the study progressed at school, her daughter asked for milk for the in-between-meal lunch at four o'clock. She overheard her daughter saying, "I have really learned a lot from that unit of work. Perhaps I shall not always act on it, but I know a lot more about foods than I ever did before. Even if I may not always observe it now, it is the kind of information one does not forget. I know that it has been useful."

One of the boys stated that:

He and his chum found the nutrition books on the Reserve Shelf in the library so interesting that they were taking home three or four each night.

A mother of an over-weight girl writes:

Balanced meals have become of vital concern to Mary. Restaurant meals are criticized and commented upon. We live in a perpetual calorie count. Mary has lost ten pounds since the work in nutrition started. I think the material covered in your work has been of great interest. We have been told at home about the experiments, and have heard many of your discussions repeated. Interest that carries beyond the class and becomes a part of everyday experience seems particularly worth while.

Another mother who deplored the fact that her daughter craved to be thin states:

I really think Sally's attitude toward food is not a typical one. She has always been food conscious because she never has been allowed to eat all she would like to. At two weeks of age she was put on a limited diet. She resents any choice of food because of its nutritive value and, because she has always been so healthy, is inclined to scoff at the idea of food for health. In fact, she longs to be anaemic.

I do think, however, that this class has made her realize the value of a balanced diet, particularly as it coincides with a class I have been taking with Dr. Rose. I believe the knowledge of food values will be very useful to her later, and her very rebellion and emotional response to discussion of food will make her remember it.

I think it is a valuable unit for children of this age.

Sally has enjoyed making her graphs, and has learned something from them. She has often made remarks such as "Spinach has almost everything in it" or "See how little, except calories, most fats have."

And from another home:

Bob has been very interested in the nutrition course. He has changed agreeably in regard to eating between meals and in eating too many sweets.

There have been discussions of calorie values at the evening meals since the course started. When I criticized my daughter for taking so much grape juice in the warm weather instead of plain water, she tried to reassure me about the energy value of grape sugar. She has repeatedly commented on the vitamin content of our diet. However, it does not seem to affect her choice of food (she still dislikes the vegetables and enjoys the starches). She is quite conscious of their relative value.

Another girl's mother writes:

My daughter calculated basal metabolic needs from three different tables instead of one, interestedly, and announced that the somewhat rough calculations were within 100 calories of each other. . . . All along she has spoken interestedly, even affectionately of the rats used in the nutrition experiments and also the other animals used for breeding experiments. She commented that she had obtained lots of practice in addition and other arithmetical processes in computing "shares." One day she said, "Don't you think I should put down that this is whole rice we are having for dinner, as that makes a difference and is important."

A slightly different note comes in:

I feel that my daughter considered this unit not quite necessary as we have always made this study of great importance at home. However, I recognize the fact that there are many young people in whose homes the well-balanced diet is stressed, and who are not as sensible about it as my daughter is and to whom this unit may be of great value.

And from other homes:

My son used to be unwilling to eat certain foods and I think had little desire for food, but has changed in this respect especially since the past few months. He says he enjoys the unit very much. Some of the work he brought home, he obviously enjoyed doing. As for myself, I think this type of science teaching is valuable and must be very interesting to the children. I should like to see some follow-up along the same idea next year. If young people can be taught how to maintain their health in adolescence, the carry-over into adulthood will bring real social gains.

I think [says Vera's mother] that the unit on the relation of diet to health is very much worth while, for through such a unit they acquire the principles of choice which will prove valuable to them. Vera has remarked that bulk of food is no evidence of calorie value. In order to give her practice in the application of these principles I plan to have her make out the menus for our family this summer.

I should like to add [writes the mother of Peter] that Peter's interest in food values has been beneficial to the entire family and made all its members calorie and vitamin conscious.

Helen prefers fruits to any other kind of dessert, but lately has shown more interest in custards and rice puddings. I would attribute both to her nutrition study. One morning recently she was served with ———. She does not care much for it, and said to me, "It has almost no energy value and doesn't do me much good." She is always asking for oatmeal.

I think that Ruth has learned a great deal about nutrition in the last few weeks, and I know that she has enjoyed the course very much. She has spoken about some of her friends being thin and pale, and she said she guessed they didn't get enough vitamins or calories. One day she said she wanted to have liver often as it was so good for her. I think that the course has been quite worth while.

Sometimes boys and girls were so interested in certain phases of the experiments that they made unique contributions, like the girl who asked if it would be possible to have X-ray pictures made of the vitamin D deficient animals. She had her father, who is a physician, plan to do it.

Three adolescent girls wished to find out the effects of coffee drinking and asked to set up a laboratory experiment to study this. Both cages of rats were fed whole wheat bread. One pair of rats was given milk to drink and the other coffee. All of these girls followed the experiment with intense interest, reporting their findings to the rest of the class as the changes took place.

Excerpt from a note-book of one pupil:

We have finished a topic on nutrition. So what? Will it be forgotten like most of the other subjects will be over the summer? It won't—at least I won't forget it. It has proved to be one of the most interesting and certainly the most useful subject we have learned this year, besides being the best thing in science I've had. I think it should prove hard forgetting what I've learned although I certainly don't intend to start "counting the calories."

One of the secretaries met a biology pupil in the hall one day and he informed her that he was so interested in the unit that he was taking it as a topic in another class. He mentioned touring Harlem in a Social Studies course, and said he was amazed to read some of the advertisements there, particularly about some mineral water which was a "cure-all." He was astonished, he said, to find so many people believe all they read in advertisements.

Some of the best evidence of worth-whileness of the experiences pupils are having is to be found in samples of their work. This work can be judged for comprehension as shown by their ability to select pertinent data, by the thoroughness of their treatment of such data, and by their organization of these data into a coherent whole. It is likewise possible to obtain evidence of pupil enthusiasm for the educational experience which in turn reflects the suitability of it for them. Two examples of pupil work during the experiment at the Lincoln School seem clearly to demonstrate this. The following report was given to the class by one of two pupils who visited the Nutrition Laboratory at Teachers College to find out what means were used to measure respiration.

We went over to Miss Bosley's office with the main idea of finding out about the Douglas bag. The Douglas bag was never used over at Teachers College because it takes so much practice to use it that if the operator does not run it regularly, he forgets how to do it. Also, it is not simple to use and not everyone can learn how to run it. It also is used by wearing a mask, and Professor McLeod believes that a mask is an inaccurate method of measurement, as the "patient" must strain somewhat, and thereby use up more energy than ordinary. It works like this: the bag is empty at first, and as the wearer breathes into it, the air collects. There is a one-way valve on it so it is just like blowing up a balloon. This collects all the expelled air, and after the test is through, the operator analyzes the gases left for carbon dioxide content.

In 1931 at Teachers College the respiration chamber was brought into use. First it was used downtown in a nursery-school. There the children played on the floor of the chamber with toys, etc. Another test was run with the children sleeping after their dinner. The next test was like this: Some steps were built to fit into the corner of the chamber. Then three girls, from 9 to 10 years of age got into the room. For twenty minutes they played quietly with books, games, etc. Then, at a given signal they started, by timing themselves with a metronome, to walk up the stairs, one by one. As there were but four stairs up and down, one girl would be on the stairs all the time.

The air is forced through a double door from the outside, in. As it comes out, it passes through several absorbers. Some of these absorbers contain soda lime to extract the carbon dioxide. Others have sulphuric acid in them, to take out the water vapor from the exhaled air which is drawn out through the bottom of the chamber.

A sample of the air in the chamber is drawn off and analyzed, the air that passed out is measured on gas meters, and the operator can figure up the oxygen consumed. Inside the chamber is sometimes placed a bicycle apparatus. This affair is really mounted on a bike frame. This machine is used to measure work spent and work received, or efficiency. Where the rear wheel should be is a copper disc. Around this is an armature which holds the disc back to some extent. On the disc a section is painted black, thus every time the light beam which is connected to a photo-electric cell hits this black section, it reflects, and generates enough electricity to move a dial, thus recording revolutions per minute. The disc is counterbalanced by a counterweight. Thus the energy output, or work, is measured by the friction of the bike chain plus the resistance of the armature plus the resistance of the counterbalance. All this is carefully computed and compared with the energy intake as measured by the methods described before. An average boy was found to be about 15 per cent efficient. The speed of pedalling is controlled by two contacts to the armature (which swings over the disc) which in turn light two lights, red and green. To maintain the proper speed, the subject must keep both lights out. The speed usually set is the average pedalling speed, 55-65 R.P.M.

All the energies are related to the basal line. However, basal metabolism is quite another story and we shall not try to explain it here. Several instruments used for taking these tests were over at Teachers College. They all worked on the same principle, which was air intake. Some were hitched up to graphs and some worked by motor, some by valves, but they all reached the same conclusions in the same way. To be accurate, one subject is given three tests on three different instruments. This is a two-way check. These instruments are made in Boston at a cost of from sixty-five dollars to two-hundred dollars. The doctors in New York working on these sorts of tests at this time (1936) are Professor McLeod, whom we interviewed, and Doctors DuBois and Bailey.

Pupils demonstrated their enjoyment in the work, and showed their ability to organize and present the outcomes they deemed valuable, by planning a dinner and an evening program for parents at the culmination of their study. At this time pupil committees suggested the menu, purchased and prepared the food, worked out an exhibit of educational materials, and wrote without assistance their talks for the program. Following are two of the many pupil speeches given:

Pupil 1. I am glad to see so many parents here this evening. I hope you are all very healthy after your vitamin dinner. Two classes have been studying science and nutrition. It seems that all our lost hopes have been prophesied for us. We expect to live happily for ever and ever. The pathetic thing about nutrition seems to be that scientists who have found out all of these things for us are too old now to benefit by this knowledge. They call on us, the youth of the country, to show what may be done. They have worked with guinea pigs. The science of nutrition, as we have been studying it this year, is a science that has sprung from almost nothing forty years ago, to a full-fledged and important science today. Its first experimenters little dreamed what wonders it had in store for them, and the world was oblivious to such things as vitamins and calories, words that now almost every food advertisement or dietitian uses in trying to scare us, perhaps justly, into health.

It was when a diet of absolutely pure food extracts was found not to support life, even though the energy value was the same as that of normal foods, that the presence of vitamins was first noticed. There must be something in the raw or natural foods that is not present in the highly refined diet. And once more these then unseen substances are essential and vital for life and growth, and hence their title, vitamins, as the scientists of twenty-five years ago named them.

Through the discovery of vitamins came also the discovery of the nutritional diseases that are caused by vitamin deficiency. And this side of nutrition built up the field of animal experimenting which has been of more help to this rapidly growing science than almost anything else.

The other aspect of nutrition deals with foods and the amount of energy they give the body. What are the energy-giving foods, and what are the foods that are mostly water and cellulose? Our body machine needs a definite amount of energy to usher it through its day of activity, and even when asleep the body is burning fuel. A vitamin diet is useless if it just consists of vitamins. The diet also must supply foods that give energy. And also the matter of bulk must come into consideration. No one expects us to eat ten heads of lettuce, that are very low in calorie content, or two or three lumps of sugar with a few vitamin pills. And so along with the vitamin content of foods, must also be found the energy value.

Food and energy are so closely tied up with heat that most of our means for determining the energy value of foods seem to use this method. The body keeps at a level temperature with only a few degrees variance due to sickness or a run-down condition. The energy that is not consumed in producing this body heat is either used up in motion and exercise or the building up of body tissues, the process of growth, and the usual functions of the body, such as the process of digestion, or the energy required in breathing or even living.

When we take food into our body, we are essentially taking in fuel, just as wood is supplied to a fire, to give us a supply of energy that we will eventually use, and there are certain chemical compounds called catalysts, especially adapted to burning or getting the energy value out of this raw material. The only way that these same foods can be turned into energy outside of the body is at temperatures no body tissue could stand, but though the temperature used in burning foods in a calorimeter, which we will study presently, is far greater than that in a human body, nevertheless the proportion is the same. And so we can burn foods in the laboratory under carefully measured conditions and get at least some approximation of the amount of energy they produce in the human body.

The energy unit that all American experimenters have used is the calorie, which is literally the amount of heat energy consumed in raising one liter of water one degree Centigrade. The simplest method of determining the calorie value of foods is with the oxy-calorimeter. A measured amount of food is placed in a container, sealed except for a safety valve, and pure oxygen is forced in around it. This inner container is further surrounded by an outer container, and there is a measured amount of water between the two separate walls. The inner container is then ignited by means of an electric spark, and with the aid of the oxygen, the food is burned. The rise in temperature in the surrounding water will naturally give an indication of the heat given off, and by knowing the amount of food burned, and by knowing the volume of water used and the amount of change in temperature, calorie values can be computed.

Well, now that we know the amount of energy foods produce in the body, the next step is to find the amount of energy the body needs, in its varied purposes throughout the day. We have already said that energy is required in producing body heat, in giving power to our muscles, when we walk, sit, breathe, even when we are asleep, but this energy need varies greatly with the individual. Weight and body surface have a great deal to do with the required energy input, and likewise age, and sex, whether one is growing or not, whether one is sick or healthy, the activities one participates in through the day, such as whether one rides in taxis or walks over country roads.

The first energy value to find is what is commonly called the basal metabolism. That is, the energy consumed when a person is spending as little energy as possible. And this is found by means of an instrument such as the Benedict's respiratory machine which we shall demonstrate.

After this basal rate is determined and the activities of the person throughout the day are found, it is possible to find out the number of calories the person tested needs. Also, if the body is not functioning perfectly, it shows up in the basal, and defects in the complicated system of the body show up in this way.

There are two or three methods of determining energy consumption and the most common of these is by measurement of the oxygen consumed in the burning process of the catalysts. Digestion is a process of oxidation, and so oxygen is naturally used up in proportion to the energy spent. The oxygen used in the burning is turned into carbon dioxide, which is exactly what, say, a candle flame will do. And so this process of oxidation gives us two methods of determining consumed energy—we can either measure the oxygen absorbed, as this apparatus here does, or measure the amount of carbon dioxide given off, in respiration. Another, and perhaps the simplest way is to measure the amount of heat a body at rest gives off and thereby measure the amount of energy used in maintaining body heat, one of the main drains of our energy supply. This method is used in the ice calorimeter which will be demonstrated in a few minutes.

[Pupil 1 then went to the board on which was a sketch of a calorimeter.

He explained the calorimeter. By measuring the rise in temperature in the surrounding water one can get an indication of heat given off.]

Pupil 10. Pupil 9 has told you about vitamin C and milk. I am going to tell you about some of the other things that are necessary in order to have good teeth of your own instead of the dentist's variety.

I am going to try to state briefly the importance of the mineral elements in nutrition. The proper amount of minerals is necessary in order to have strong rigid bones and teeth. They are essential to the body fluids. Muscles and nerves must be bathed and nourished by fluid containing the right proportions of salts and certain mineral elements. The rhythmic contraction and relaxation of the heart muscles which constitutes the beating of the heart is dependent upon the presence of the right proportions of calcium, sodium, and potassium.

You have all been told to eat spinach, for it contains iron. But the amazing thing is you actually need iron, for the red blood corpuscles are conspicuously dependent for their normal composition and function upon the iron which they contain. Iron is essential in the manufacturing of new red blood corpuscles. Cases of anaemia are due to the absence of a sufficient amount of iron to form new red corpuscles. Anaemia lessens the resistance to disease and causes one to be lackadaisical and tired. Most green leafy vegetables are rich in the important mineral elements.

The body needs a greater amount of calcium and phosphorous than any other mineral matter. At least 99 per cent of the calcium and over two-thirds of the phosphorous which the body contains is found in the bones and teeth.

Potassium and sulphur are fairly prominent among the essential mineral elements in the body. If your diet contains a sufficient amount of calcium, phosphorous and iron, present knowledge indicates that it will contain enough of the other mineral elements which the body needs.

The body requires many different minerals. When you hear the list, don't think you are listening to a mining engineer, rather realize that all these elements are essential to human development.

In addition to iron, calcium, phosphorous, potassium and sulphur, the body also needs sodium, chlorine, magnesium, copper, manganese, and iodine. All these minerals need not trouble you, for if you get a mixed diet, there will be a sufficient amount of these minerals present to keep you healthy and contribute to a long life.

We used to pay most attention to our calcium intake. Children who receive a rich supply of calcium and phosphorous in their diet have a much better chance of having healthy teeth and strong bones.

Compared with the composition of a normal adult, the body of a child at birth is iron rich and calcium poor. This condition is normal, because if a body had a lot of calcium in his bones they would be hard, and he would probably kill his mother when being born. Hence, it is extremely important for a child to have a liberal intake of calcium in order to compensate for its insufficient amount at birth. One of the best ways of getting a sufficient amount of calcium is to drink 4 cups of milk a day.

To insure an adequate supply of calcium, eat proper amounts of the foods you see on display.

APPRAISAL BY PARTICIPATING TEACHERS

At the close of the investigation the cooperating teachers were asked to discuss the experiment in terms of its value to the pupils, its value to them as teachers, the difficulties encountered, and their plan for improving the organization of the teaching materials.

Teacher 1 in School A reports:

The animal feeding experiment was most significant. The experience of the guinea pig that lost weight so rapidly from lack of Vitamin C and finally had an intestinal hemorrhage, and then with the application of Vitamin C, recovered so quickly—carried weight with the class. Charts took on more meaning when supplemented by this experience. . . . We added an experiment that indicated that soda lime takes up CO_2. . . . One copy of such books as Sherman's *Food and Health* is inadequate for class needs.

Teacher 2 in School A reports:

A biology course is not fully complete without a good study of the relationship of diet and health to the human body. To do this effectively, the use of animals is necessary. The only fault I found with this unit was the extra time it would take. A person could spend one semester in this one unit as here outlined. In general biology two weeks is usually all we find time for food study.

As for the unit itself, it is very complete and worked so each point is well developed. One part leads up logically to the next point in a very interesting way.

A teacher in School B reports he is decidedly enthusiastic about the experiment, which challenged him to do the best teaching he has ever done. He added much reference material, constructed supplementary tests, and had pupils conduct numerous laboratory experiments on the relation of chemistry to nutrition.

A teacher in School C used comments of the pupils to evaluate the study:

The work in this unit is very interesting to me. The laboratory animals enable us to understand more clearly the object of the unit, the value of nutrition.

The study of vitamins and calories is worthy of our attention, and the knowledge obtained will be valuable to us especially in the future when we have homes of our own.

Basal metabolism, although difficult, was one of the most interesting parts of the unit. I like the problems now, although at first I could not do them correctly.

The only parts of the whole unit that I did not like were the tests. We are not used to those types of tests, but with very few exceptions we have direct questions or matching columns.

It was during this study that I had my only connection with experiments on laboratory animals. These provided entertainment, and yet demonstrated even to a fuller extent than books, the fundamentals which we were driving at. The experiments with the respiration apparatus, using our classmates as the guinea pigs, clearly showed the use of the instrument; and how our energy needs are determined.

I believe the books by Sherman and Rose were too difficult for tenth-year science pupils. However, I did enjoy the unit and know that the boys and girls did also. Several times they expressed the idea that they were getting more worthwhile material, applicable to their everyday life, than in any other subject.

Teacher 1 in School D reports: "We found the unit interesting and profitable."

Teacher 2 in School D reports:

In general, the students were quite interested in the entire unit. It took several days to get them in the right attitude, but once there, it seemed to last. I heartily agree that the unit should carry some animal experimentation. The duller members of the classes seemed to come out and shine in this part of the work. The experiments were in charge of a junior girl who plans to take up diet work when she graduates from high school. Working with her were six or seven others selected from the various sections. . . . We encountered a cold spell during the vacation and the temperature of the biology lab became quite low. The two low calorie rats and one vitamin rat passed on—died! Thus demonstrating the need for food to keep the body at living temperature. Rather a short experiment we thought! We immediately split up the rats again putting one to the cage instead of two, and started the experiments again. The entire experiment, with cages, animals, scales, food and students was photographed and printed in an issue of the school paper. . . . Unless the results from the tests were surprising, I still feel that the general language level of the tests were somewhat above the general word knowledge of the biology students. They seem to be weak in their knowledge of word meaning and use. . . . I was sorry to find that you had not indicated any slides, film slides, or motion pictures as a part of the work. I have in mind the Department of Agriculture's picture, "Food

Makes a Difference"; the Y.M.C.A. films, "Food and Growth," "Good Foods—Bread and Cereals"; "The Amazing Vitamins" and "Vitamin Secrets Revealed." The sound films by Erpi, "Digestion," "Distribution of Foods," and the "Heart and Circulation of Blood." I mention this because you seem to have provided for several of the other types of visual aids—charts, graphs, and pictures.

A teacher in School E reports:

I feel very grateful to you for giving me the opportunity of trying the project in my school. The illustrative material, charts, and references are very valuable as an aid in starting the unit.

The interest has been very good during all of the project. Some of the activities we have included are experiments on ice calorimeter (homemade), water calorimeter (homemade), respiration calorimeter (same as yours), animal experiments including rats, guinea pigs, and pigeons. Each member of the class analyzed one kind of food for water content, ash, and combined carbohydrates, fat, and protein. A composite was made of all data.

Our animal experiments were very positive in results, both in growth and in healthy characteristics.

A teacher in School F reports: [3]

I still feel the Sherman book is not satisfactory as a high-school text. I very much like *Foundations of Nutrition.*

The rats on the low-calorie diet were found dead Monday morning. This was due to the janitor's failure to take care of them over the weekend. I tried to drive the lesson home, that girls who starve themselves to retain boyish figures are apt to meet with tragedy in the case of an emergency.

I am very much discouraged with the respiration apparatus. Evidently I have not sufficient training in handling mechanical difficulties that arise. The boys in the class have been most helpful and resourceful.

This teacher listed certain favorable and unfavorable reactions:

1. The use of the live animals vitalized the work.
2. Care of the animals by boys who otherwise have difficulty in handling the subject gave them an opportunity to show their real interest in the subject. It gave me a much higher opinion of these students.
3. The boys enjoyed their efforts in making cages, and in surmounting the difficulties encountered in making the respiration apparatus work. As most of the students were boys, interest ran high.
4. The effort to secure aid for books brought us, as a class, more closely together. The Chemistry, Physics, Forging, Student Council, Refec-

[3] Accidentally the raw scores of tests from this school were destroyed, and hence data are not included from School F.

tory, and Home Economics Departments all helped us. Hence, the goal of integration in education was approximated.

5. My own unfamiliarity with the unit made me feel inadequate and clumsy. A second effort, I feel sure, would bring better results and greater happiness.
6. Much too complicated for the majority of our students. Poor students had to be helped over and over in the making of the energy calculations, and then could not apply their knowledge on tests.

She also stated:

The work has helped me to see the need of making my work more concrete, and has aided in suggesting ways of making Biology less bookish, and giving students more opportunities to show abilities other than fact accumulation.

A teacher in School G reports:

In this school no animal experimentation was carried on, nor was the respiration apparatus used. There was difficulty in maintaining interest of boys and girls in the work, which seems to reflect the difficulty of teaching without laboratory experiences. . . . I still hope to do some work in trying out your unit as I know how worthwhile it is.

A teacher in School H reports:

The animal experiment was enjoyed by all and most of the results were good. Our homemade respiration apparatus gave only fair results, as a result of poor construction, yet the boys and girls enjoyed working with it, and with a few improvements it will remain a permanent part of our laboratory equipment.

Additional experiments: Pupils tested per cent of hemoglobin in their own blood by the use of color charts and made and stained blood smears.

I believe the unit serves a much-needed function in schools where a full year's course in nutrition is not taught, in that it gives a much-needed knowledge of foods and their relation to health. I know of nowhere else the majority of my group would be given this training. The unit also ties up the processes of digestion, assimilation, respiration, and circulation which are often-times considered by biologists in too isolated a fashion.

SUMMARY

The data from the first experiment at the Lincoln School showed that the pupils made significant gains in each of the attributes measured.

The retention tests given a year later showed that the pupils in the experimental matched group had retained all gains made in the attitudes test and in the application of principles test, and three-fourths of the gains made on the information test.

The data from the extended experiment showed that in all cases where pupils were not under serious handicap, the groups made significant gains in their attitude toward the selection of diet, in information about the relation of food to health, and in all but one of the instances in the application of principles.

The low intercorrelations between the tests indicate that each measures a separate attribute and that pupils at this level of maturity do not achieve the integrated understanding held by experts; the lower intercorrelations between the final tests indicate that the pupils are progressing along divergent lines or at different rates.

The samples of pupil work cited indicate the extent to which pupils may progress in understanding fundamental concepts having to do with the relation of food to physical well-being.

The records given by parents indicate that pupils are carrying some of the understandings into their everyday lives and practicing them in relation to their own welfare.

The appraisal by the various participating teachers indicates that they felt the organization a most useful one, as well as one dealing with functional materials which better enabled the pupils to solve their everyday problems.

CHAPTER VI

Summary of the Investigation

THE author undertook this investigation because of his conviction that something should be done to aid adolescents to understand and use recent knowledge of nutrition in the selection of their daily diet. Adolescents show in their questions a driving interest in those things which vitally affect them. They are maturing rapidly and habits of action established by them during this period are likely to persist throughout life. The newer knowledge of nutrition indicates that the general level of efficiency and well-being could be considerably raised by attention to the daily intake of food. Science education is particularly concerned with adequate health instruction, and nutrition is an important part of this instruction.

The problem was stated, "Can the study of the relation of food to physical well-being, in high school biology classes, be truly educative?" The solution of this problem depended upon whether or not the outcomes could be detected and measured, and whether or not the outcomes were such that they function in the daily lives of the pupils.

The procedure used was to select and organize the educational experiences for use in biology classes; to select the attributes for measurement and construct valid and reliable tests for their measurement; to plan situations for securing descriptive means of evaluation in the form of anecdotal records and an appraisal by other teachers using the material; and to provide experimental situations where the changes made by high school pupils studying nutrition could be studied.

The first experiment was conducted at the Lincoln School of Teachers College. Stenographic reports of behavior and the opportunity to retest a year after the close of the instruction were possible in this situation. The extended experiment included different teachers in varying situations. These included two private schools in New York City and eight selected schools in the New Jersey, Pennsylvania, Delaware, and Ohio. The population of the towns in which these schools were situated ranged from a few hundred to over four hundred thousand.

In the first experiment the teaching was done by the investigator with the cooperation and guidance of the school home economics teacher and a graduate student in nutrition. Especial effort was made to collect descriptive evidence of pupil reactions. An experimental group and a control group of ninth and tenth graders were selected. Initial tests were given at the beginning of the experimental period, final tests at the end of the experimental period, and retention tests a year after the instruction ceased.

In the extended experiment, the organization was carefully rewritten, many specific suggestions for teaching were added, and help was given in the preparation of diets and the securing of animals and other equipment essential to the unit. The same test forms were given at the beginning and at the end of the experimental period. Two teachers in one school cooperated by giving the tests without instruction in nutrition during the interim. This provided a measure of the practice effect from taking the tests, and the matching of equivalent groups for a comparison of the gains made.

The findings of the investigation showed that the study of the relation of food to physical well-being was truly educative in that as a result of instruction, pupils in varying types of school situations made significant gains in their attitude toward food in diet, in their information concerning the relation of food to physical well-being, and in their application of nutrition principles in the interpretation of food advertisements. Selected samples of pupil work illustrate a high degree of interest and understanding achieved as a result of the educational experiences. Statements from parents further indicate that pupils do use knowledge gained from this study as a basis for action in their daily lives. The appraisal of the educational experiences by the participating teachers gives their testimony as to the worth of such experiences in high school biology classes.

The first experiment at Lincoln School revealed that pupils retain most of the gains made when tested one year after the experimental period. Study of all pupils from the first experimental situation shows that roughly all of the gains made in attitude, two-thirds of the gains made in information, and one-half of the gains made in the application of nutrition principles are retained after the duration of one year. When compared, the two equivalent groups of fifteen pupils each, matched in age, intelligence, and initial test scores, show that after an interval of a year the pupils having the instruction retained all gains made in attitudes and in application of principles, but lost about one-fourth of the gain in information. The equivalent group which did not have such instruction rated slightly lower on each retention test than on each initial test. Therefore, practice effect had no appreciable influence on the test results.

That effective application of this organization of educational experiences can be made in various kinds of schools by biology teachers is shown in several ways. The experiments suggested proved stimulating and workable. The use of animals resulted in interest and understanding not otherwise possible. Study of nutrition in biology classes resulted in teacher growth, and indicated ways to make the biology curriculum more functional. The fact that two schools did not make significant gains can be readily accounted for by their serious handicap in lack of reference material.

The interest and enthusiasm of adolescents, together with their use of understandings achieved in their daily selection of diet and in their interpretation of food advertisements, show that this work does help them meet their needs.

The low intercorrelations between the attributes measured in either the initial or the final tests indicate that the tests used measure different attributes and that the pupils did not progressively gain at the same rate in each of these attributes.

INTERPRETATIONS

The cooperating teachers demonstrated that the educational experiences basic to this investigation[1] provide an organization for use in high school classes.

Adolescents are interested in this way of studying nutrition, and since it is in line with the objectives of education, one feels confident that such opportunities for study should be provided in the high school curriculum. Since laboratory experiences are essential it seems advisable to include this work in the general biology course.

[1] Cf. Chapter II.

Reference materials, texts, and illustrative material for use in this unit are as yet relatively inaccessible.

A number of participating teachers felt—it seems wisely—that use should be made of available movie films related to the study of nutrition.

Pupils have often expressed the opinion that this study has more connection between their daily lives than any other phase of the curriculum.

Anecdotal records[2] give evidence that pupils need concrete experiences, such as animal experimentation, use of respiration apparatus, analysis of ash content of foods, and the like, to gain interests, understandings, and appreciations capable of functioning in their daily lives.

Biology teachers should accept responsibility for instruction of adolescents in the relation of food to their physical well-being.

Opportunities and experiences which will make prospective teachers alert and responsive in adapting the curriculum to the needs of adolescent boys and girls should be provided during the teacher-training period.

More evidence is needed regarding the extent to which pupils integrate classroom experiences, and methods of teaching which facilitate such integration.

This study has shown how materials of vital importance to boys and girls can be so organized and taught that they function in their daily lives. It seems that other problems closely related to human welfare, such as personal hygiene, safety, control of disease, sex, recreation, and psychology, might yield fruitful results if studied somewhat after the pattern used in this investigation.

[2] Cf. Chapter IV.

Bibliography

BOOKS—GENERAL

FISHER, R. A. *Statistical Methods for Research Workers.* Oliver and Boyd, Edinburgh, 1937.

GARRETT, H. E. *Statistics in Psychology and Education.* (Revised Edition.) Longmans, Green and Company, New York, 1937.

GUILFORD, I. P. *Psychometric Methods.* McGraw-Hill Book Company, New York, 1936.

KELLEY, T. L. *Interpretation of Educational Measurement.* World Book Company, Yonkers-on-Hudson, N. Y., 1927.

MCCALL, W. A. *How to Experiment in Education.* The Macmillan Company, New York, 1926.

ROBERTS, L. J. *Nutrition Work with Children.* (Second Edition.) University of Chicago Press, Chicago, Ill., 1936.

ROSE, M. S. *Foundations of Nutrition.* The Macmillan Company, New York, 1935.

ROSE, M. S. *Teaching Nutrition to Boys and Girls.* The Macmillan Company, New York, 1932.

SHERMAN, H. C. *Food and Health.* The Macmillan Company, New York, 1935.

STARCH, DAVID. *Educational Psychology.* The Macmillan Company, New York, 1928.

SYMONDS, P. M. *Measurement in Secondary Education.* The Macmillan Company, New York, 1927.

THURSTONE, L. L. *The Reliability and Validity of Tests.* Edwards Brothers, Ann Arbor, Michigan, 1931.

THURSTONE, L. L. AND CHAVE, E. J. *Measurement of Attitude.* University of Chicago Press, Chicago, Ill., 1929.

PERIODICALS

MITCHELL, D. C. "A Survey of Health Instruction in Senior High Schools." *The Research Quarterly of the American Physical Education Association,* Vol. 5, No. 3, Oct., 1934, pp. 127-135.

RATHS, L. E. *Evaluating the Ability of Students to Apply Facts, Definitions, and Principles.* Evaluation in the Eight Year Study, Progressive Education Association, Bulletin 5, Dec., 1936, p. 2.

REMINGTON, R. E. "The Social Origins of Dietary Habits." *Scientific Monthly,* Vol. XVIII, Sept., 1936, pp. 193-204.

THURSTONE, L. L. "Attitudes Can Be Measured." *American Journal of Sociology,* Vol. 33, 1928, pp. 529-554.

TYLER, R. W. "Techniques Evaluating Behavior." *Educational Research Bulletin* (Ohio State University), Jan. 17, 1934, pp. 1-11.

MONOGRAPHS AND REPORTS

SHERMAN, H. C. *Nutritional Improvement in Health and Longevity.* Supplementary Publications No. 25. Issued by Carnegie Institution of Washington, Office of Publications, Washington, D. C., Aug. 15, 1936.

NATIONAL SOCIETY FOR THE STUDY OF EDUCATION. *Thirty-First Year Book,* Part I. Public School Publishing Co., Bloomington, Ill., 1932.

UNITED STATES BUREAU OF EDUCATION. *Cardinal Principles of Secondary Education.* Bulletin No. 35, 1918. Superintendent of Document, Washington, D. C., 1918.

UNITED STATES BUREAU OF EDUCATION. *Organization of Science in the Secondary Schools,* Bulletin No. 26, 1920. p. 11.

THESES

CAIRNS, LAURA. *A Scientific Basis for Health Instruction in Public Schools.* Ph.D. Thesis, University of California Press, Berkeley, Cal., 1929.

STATISTICAL TABLES

HOLZINGER, K. J. *Statistical Tables for Students in Education and Psychology.* University of Chicago Press, Chicago, Ill., 1931.

SNEDECOR, G. W. *Statistical Methods.* Collegiate Press, Inc., Ames, Iowa, 1937.